RAPID WEIGHT LOSS HYPNOSIS

The Effective Method of Losing Weight Healthily in Less Than 10 Days. Learn To Eat Mindfully Through Meditation and Simple Habits. Increase Your Self-Esteem Easily

By

Dave Carnegie

© **Copyright 2020 All rights reserved.**

This document is geared towards providing exact and reliable information with regards to the topic and issue covered. The publication is sold with the idea that the publisher is not required to render accounting, officially permitted, or otherwise, qualified services. If advice is necessary, legal or professional, a practiced individual in the profession should be ordered.

From a Declaration of Principles which was accepted and approved equally by a Committee of the American Bar Association and a Committee of Publishers and Associations.

In no way is it legal to reproduce, duplicate, or transmit any part of this document in either electronic means or in printed format. Recording of this publication is strictly prohibited and any storage of this document is not allowed unless with written permission from the publisher. All rights reserved.

The information provided herein is stated to be truthful and consistent, in that any liability, in terms of inattention or otherwise, by any usage or abuse of any policies, processes, or directions contained within is the solitary and utter responsibility of the recipient reader. Under no circumstances will any legal responsibility or blame be held against the publisher for any reparation, damages, or monetary loss due to the information herein, either directly or indirectly.

Respective authors own all copyrights not held by the publisher. The information herein is offered for informational purposes solely, and is universal as so. The presentation of the information is without contract or any type of guarantee assurance.

Table of Contents

INTRODUCTION

There are many weight-loss options in today's modern world that we can use. Some commercials or videos promise to help you lose weight quickly. You can also come across advertisements on TVs that give you a fast weight loss and how to get the body you want in a short time. They lavish us with all kinds of goods and pills, and most of them tell us they have the fastest way to get rid of excess pounds quickly. They have generated many disturbances and can also sell diets, drugs, workout equipment, and workout plans.

Our eating habits are affected by our desires, our feelings, our values, and our emotions. Both of these are under the influence of our subconscious minds. The subconscious mind trains us to maintain a certain level of weight, and we will continue to consume the amount of food required to sustain us at that level. All this is done automatically, and we're going to eat less, we're going to weigh less. We must always reprogram our subconscious mind to eat less and use our subconscious power to believe, look, and think like a lean person. If we successfully do this, our eating habits will change, and we can achieve accelerated weight loss, natural weight loss, and healthy weight loss.

In this book, you will get to deepen your understanding of the easy way to lose weight in less than ten days. You can also improve your self-esteem quickly and learn to eat thoughtfully through simple routines and meditation. You would be able to attain your ideal balanced and enviable body and also benefit from self-hypnosis in achieving weight loss. You will hear about the step-by-step guide to achieving weight loss naturally and easily. In the next chapter, we will begin to understand the mind through hypnosis.

CHAPTER ONE

HOW DOES THE MIND WORK?

It's always an excellent idea to have an idea of how the mind functions to change your sales copy differently to cater to those mind sectors. Let's just start with some simple details, so you get a clear idea of how your mind functions.

The brain does two important things-storing information in your memory and processing information that helps you to use/apply your knowledge to make decisions and solve problems. First, we'll look at what side of the brain is doing.

Your left brain deals with reasoning, phrases, sections and details, a thorough analysis of circumstances, and sequential thought. Interestingly enough, the left brain has a sense of time and a sense of intently connected to your role in specific objectives. Speak to me about a finely tuned instrument. The left brain governs/runs the right side of the body, too.

Your right brain deals with thoughts, images, wholes, and how all the pieces connect, bringing things together (that AH-HA moment) and a simultaneous/holistic view. This side of the brain does not wear a watch as the left side does, and it may actually lose track of time. Like the left side of the brain, the left side of your body is controlled by the right side.

Brain functions can be further broken down into what each side of the brain does to operate wisely. So, let's have a more in-depth view of what the left side is doing.

The left side of the brain deals with tasks such as logical, sequential, analytical, objective, concentration and information, and numbers. So, if you happen to be low in math, blame the left side of your brain-or the right side for not controlling the number portion of you.

The right side of the brain responsible for activities such as being intuitive. Trust your bitches, man. Typically, they are based on facts filed just below the conscious level. It also deals with colors, rhythm, and the overall picture, with images, and is random.

We've all heard about short attention span and advertisement that often seems to be the norm for consumers. What this implies is that only part of your memory can be accessed at any time, and a single region would be placed in the most easily accessed portion of your memory. It will also be the most familiar one, the one most commonly used. The more frequently it is seen, the more familiar it becomes. Think of a repetitive marketing campaign, top-of-the-line recognition, copy designed to cater to those senses that become recognizable to your consumer over time. People need to be told about a particular product or service at least seven times before they buy/try it. Think of the frequent customers here.

We spoke a little earlier about mental patterns in this book and Neuro-Linguistic Programming. Mental habits essentially refer to memories that have been formed in your brain to document your experiences as you see, hear, sound, smell, sound, or taste. The more times you do this, the brain is creating a familiar pattern.

When you witness a scenario or something similar again, the memory will be triggered, and you will be on the autopilot. So, you can see if you've done an email campaign to blend with your website copy and all the other areas we've outlined where you can use keywords and phrases, the more people see it (website or email, etc.), the more familiar you become. This way goes straight back to the marketing partnership. Is it not a cool tie in?

Okay, now you've got a pretty good understanding of how the mind works. Let's just take another step further. You already know that brain language is images, sounds, feelings, tastes, and smells-in other words, the input of your senses that is your imagination when it is processed. Your brain can only work with the positive information it receives from your five senses. Your mind can't work with inputs that you haven't experienced or otherwise called negative information.

When thinking about your clients, here is a significant thing to consider. At the same time, they can't represent and behave. They need to concentrate on one or another item (reading a copy of your website, email, etc.) and think about it or take action and purchase something. The trick is that you can quickly and efficiently move them from one to the other. Ok, you know a little deal about Neuro-Linguistic Programming and how the mind functions.

Now you know that the brain is divided into two hemispheres, each specializing in different tasks, processing different types of information, and coping with various issues—the left works with reasoning and analysis, the right with thoughts and imagination.

Let's put that in perspective as we think of our clients. And here's why you want to see what they're doing for a living thing. The manager will be a left-handed person (appeal to his / her reasoning and love of analysis). The leader will be the right brain (an appeal to his / her feelings and imagination). A producer-that will depend on the kind of work that has been done. If the work is done is logical, verbal, and analytical, the brain is left behind. If the job is intuitive, emotional, and imaginative, that's the right brain. Can you be a mix of that? Yeah, but typically one is more prevalent than the other.

The Theory of the Mind Works

Consider short-term memory as a glass of water, empty and ready to drink water (like knowledge). You slowly fill a glass with water from a fountain (a fountain of knowledge) until it is finished. But you're already serving, and the water is pouring over the edge and wasting. Short-term memory is the source of information from the efforts of research. After a while, it's complete; any more analysis is wasted. In most cases, you can take about 40-45 minutes to obtain new information. This way means that research or re-examining for longer is a waste (Practical and physical learning can and will often allow longer periods before saturation is reached, but study at the desk of any media follows this time scale).

Luckily, there is also a water storage tank (Long-term memory). You should put water in here and get it out if you want to drink it in the future. So just before the glass is full, you're going to stop filling it and dump it into the storage tank. Then you can go back to another glass and pass it to the tank as well.

What this means to research and revise is that we should prepare it in a short period, but there is another factor, and that is how successful we are in recalling information from our long-term memory. The three most effective ways to bring data into long-term memory in a way that improves the chances of survival when you want it to be:

- New: The newer the information is kept, the more likely you are to recall it.

- Frequency: The more often you repeat the information stored, the more likely you will recall it.

- Intensity: The more intense the memory-laying experience, the more likely you are to recall it.

You have the part of your mind called a conscious mind; this part is used to make decisions. You're deciding on what you're doing with your body. You often choose to think about the feelings you feel about yourself. Your conscious mind is like a gatekeeper to your subconscious mind. It can accept or reject any information provided to it. You can think of the thoughts you want to think of, and you can use your imagination to feel the emotions you want to feel.

If you want to focus on some specific topic, you can shut out any distractions that can lead you astray.

The subconscious mind is somewhat different from that of the conscious mind. Then it cannot approve or deny something.

It's just room. It will store any knowledge obtained by the conscious mind. Well, that's the secret. Your subconscious can't keep learning if your conscious mind doesn't let it go. All emotions associated with a particular scent, sound, touch, taste, and memory are in your subconscious mind. The compilations of all these memories establish the patterns you do regularly. When you are faced with new knowledge, you rely on your subconscious to decide how to behave based on past behavior references. Whether or not it's the right thing to do, your subconscious doesn't care; it's just giving you details from the past.

So, the breakdown is just like this:

The emotions that you have and the decisions that you make are all a direct product of what you have embraced in the past. What you believe is what you have gone over to your subconscious, and then it is processed with all the other knowledge in it.

This way is a good part of it; you should dismiss something that doesn't sit well.

Any negative information can be thrown away at will, and you will begin to build up the stock of only optimistic and optimistic knowledge in your subconscious mind. Once you've got this to draw on, it will be mirrored in your actions.

How would you behave today if you had positive memories? I think the sky is the limit. Leave the past where it is now. If you have a memory that's bad and doesn't suit you, don't think about it. If they're sneaking on you, quickly replace them with a happy one. You don't need the old negative baggage anyway. What's the point of going over it in your mind if you know it's going to reflect on your actions? Know, there's no job you can't do in the past. You won't be able to function in the future because it is not here. You can only work right now. Your acts will be replicated in the form of habits, and your actions will come as a guide to what is in your subconscious.

What is Hypnosis?

Hypnosis is a very straightforward and easy-to-explain psychological phenomenon, but it is often falsely interpreted as some form of black magic or false mysticism. This lack of equal representation leaves many to set aside "hypnotic knowledge" as mere illusion or hogwash, and those who have been hypnotized are usually considered to be weak-minded or gullible. But none of this is real.

Before I continue with the debunking of these myths, let me first offer a brief description of what hypnosis is:

Hypnosis is a collection of powerful communication strategies (often with overt or indirect "suggestions") to influence one's values, emotions, feelings, and behaviors.

Despite this broad definition, this is what hypnosis is all about. Let's get started now.

MYTH 1: Hypnosis is a state of perception

Hypnosis is not linked to any actual state of consciousness at all. The reason people confuse hypnosis with a state of consciousness because we frequently equate hypnosis methods with half-sleep and half-awakening. We imagine patients lying on leather sofas with their eyes closed and their consciousness facing inward to their "subconscious." But the truth is that hypnosis can be used to raise awareness just as easily as it can be used to contract awareness.

The best example of hypnosis in "natural" consciousness is stage hypnosis. When a person clucks like a chicken or performs a scene in Saving Private Ryan, it's not because the individual is unconscious and is pulled by his or her strings like a stuffed puppet. They're just in a position where they're comfortable acting out actions because usually wouldn't be done in front of the audience. They're not being "mediated" by the hypnotist-they're being communicated effectively. Participants are also in touch during the whole session. A person can get his or her self out of hypnosis anytime they want, but why would they want to play when they're having so much fun?

MYTH 2: All hypnosis is "playing to pretend."

During stage hypnosis, participants are fully aware that they are not chickens or are not in the movies. They know they're acting (it so happens that hypnosis can turn people into good actors).

But not all hypnosis can be called "playing pretend." It depends on the quality of the suggestions made. If a request is to "press like a chicken," then the patient can behave. If the idea is "think about a time in your history when you felt confident"-it's not playing pretend-the patient thinks about it and connects himself with the time when they were confident.

I agree with hypnotists, who say all hypnosis is self-hypnosis. This way means that a hypnotist can't usually manipulate someone into doing something against his own will. Compliance is often found on both sides of the relationship. The only difference is that hypnotists will elicit odd or uncommon behaviors if they find the correct mode of communication.

MYTH 3: Empirical studies say that only 5 % of the population is prone to hypnosis.

This way is partially right: research reports also say that only 5-10 percent of the population is prone to hypnosis. However, these experiments are mostly inaccurate because researchers only assess subjects with traditional hypnotic inductions and standardized hypnosis scripts. Hypnosis does not operate in a one-size-fits-all fashion, though (because its strength comes from using our own personal and special connections and interpretation of language).

A proper hypnotist can read his patient, to step away from generic texts, and to discover the language most suggestive of that particular patient.

There are also techniques in NLP (Neurolinguistic Programming-a method that may be called "modern-day hypnosis") that allow NLP practitioners to discover the language patterns of an individual (sometimes referred to as "trance words" or "keywords") only by asking the patient a series of questions.

In other terms, with the right hypnotist and the right communication-anyone is predictive of hypnosis.

MYTH 4: Hypnosis is close to meditation;

This way is a common misconception. Again-hypnosis is a series of communication strategies, whereas meditation is a more personal activity that is more closely related to one's state of consciousness or mindfulness.

However, hypnosis techniques can be used to help meditative practice. What is sometimes referred to as "Guided Meditation" could be considered a form of hypnosis. A degree of self-hypnosis (i.e., no instruction from third parties) could also be used to extend or contract consciousness in a specific meditative state.

But again, hypnosis is not about a personal mental state-its about the expression of thoughts or suggestions.

At times, a specific mental state can be more conducive to learning. That's why the hypnotherapist always prefers to calm their patients before joining the bulk of their session. Comfortable people also feel more refreshed, can focus more, develop their cognitive skills, and are thus better learners.

Stage hypnotists, however, do not want to place their participants in comfortable states. That would have been a boring presentation. Instead, they typically want to instill some suspense or a sense of adventure-similar to a child's mood.

MYTH 5: Hypnosis on the highway

Hypnosis on the highway, as described by Wikipedia, says

Highway hypnosis is defined as a mental state in which a person may drive a truck or a car long distances, react to external events in an anticipated manner, without any recollection of having done so consciously. In this state, the driver's conscious mind is entirely concentrated elsewhere, with the seemingly direct processing of the masses of information required to drive safely. 'Highway Hypnosis' is only one manifestation of relatively normal experience, potentially where conscious and subconscious minds seem to be focused on various things; staff doing basic and routine tasks and sleepless individuals are likely to experience similar symptoms. It's a kind of "driving mode" subconscious.

Again, you might already be able to guess what's wrong with this definition: hypnosis is not a mental condition!

Highway hypnosis is a trance state (a change away from "everyday" awareness). There is no contact and, therefore-no, no hypnosis. Another similar trance state is when you get so absorbed in a film that you lose track of time.

It is easy to understand how these states can be confused with hypnosis because hypnosis typically likes to mimic these trance states to make them more suggestive (but remember: if there is no suggestion to communicate, not hypnosis).

MYTH 6: Hypnosis is not a genuine catalyst for physical or chemical changes in the body.

In fact, except for the simple fact that the brain is made up of electro-chemicals called neurons, which fire between 50-200 times per second, everything makes it a possible trigger for a chemical shift in the body. What we need to do is think about something and change the chemistry in our brains.

But more technically, people want to know whether hypnosis will potentially lead to improvements in the body, such as weight gain/decrease, muscle building, or even an improvement in the size of the breast/penis. Usually, the answer to all these questions is "yes, to some degree."

Hypnosis can't allow the body to do stuff; it's already unable to do spontaneously independently.

Remember: hypnosis helps make improvements to your body's full potential-it does not encourage you to overcome your biological nature via any "mystical fashion." Although there is a fair possibility that hypnosis may disclose information about your body that you previously did not know about.

MYTH 7: You should not attempt hypnosis without a professional hypnotist or hypnotherapist.

Many qualified hypnotists and hypnotherapists will advise you that you should always be a professional. But it would be so unfair of me to say that because I am self-taught, you have to do this. In reality, I believe that everyone can teach themselves a little hypnosis to check out and see the potential for themselves.

Hypnosis is a natural phenomenon-it is your natural right to explore it and explore the mind/body as a whole. There are several podcasts, books, and videos to get you started hypnosis-experiment with as many people as you want, make a difference in methods, and begin to explore the basic concepts of what makes a hypnotic versatile and successful.

Types of Hypnosis

There are still the same concepts of hypnosis by which the technique is used, but there are different pathways to do it. Certain approaches are as old as hypnosis, while others are the result of research and new techniques have therefore been developed. The form of hypnosis typically depends on the outcome that is desired. They all have their meaning, and the learning of each one opens the doors to other methods. Here are some of the key types:

Modern Hypnosis:

Traditional hypnosis is a classic hypnosis style that has been around for a long time. It is a variant of a hypnotist that puts the subject in a deep trance and then guides it by using suggestions and commands. This technique is used for stage hypnotism.

The conventional form of hypnosis has been much maligned and mocked over the years, often unjustified, but sadly some of the criticism is right. The use of fake hypnosis using stage plants and actors has weakened the conventional form of hypnosis. Applied correctly, this is a valuable and efficient tool that can be both enjoyable and helpful.

Hypnotherapy

The use of hypnosis to facilitate recovery or positive growth in some way is known as hypnotherapy. It is generally used to deal with psychological issues inside the mind, as this is where hypnosis can be powerful. Effective hypnotherapy can reprogram patterns of behavior within reason and allow things like phobias, irrational fears, addictions, and negative emotions to be regulated. Hypnotherapy can also control pain stimuli, and hypnosis has been used to perform surgery on fully conscious patients. They would be in apparent discomfort if not for the use of hypnosis.

Hypnosis can be used to support people. Hypnotherapy is used to encourage spiritual growth and facilitate recovery. Hypnotherapy can be particularly helpful for psychological disorders, such as depression. Phobias, addictions, and all sorts of irrational thoughts can be selectively reprogrammed and controlled by negative emotions. Hypnosis, as used in hypnotherapy, can also have physical consequences, the most evident being pain blocking, which enables surgical operations to be done without damage and complications associated with anesthesia.

Hypnotherapy typically uses only very mild hypnosis, not the intense trance condition used in the conventional type. Most patients are completely awake and fully aware of this. The crucial point of hypnotherapy is that the patient must stay entirely focused on treatment and listen to the words of the therapist. It is essential to maintain a good relationship with the therapist. If the patient has no confidence in or feels that the treatment will not succeed, it will fail. However, if the patient is optimistic and open-minded, the success rate is very high.

Self-hypnosis / auto-hypnosis

As the name suggests, this approach relies on the topic of self-inducing hypnosis. This approach is accomplished by studying a series of protocols or by listening to a tape. Most self-hypnosis is offered as hypnotherapy and is close to deep relaxation and meditation.

Hypnosis and self-hypnosis are somewhat similar. The main difference is that the topic is operating with the ideas rather than someone else's. It is commonly held that all hypnosis is, in fact, self-hypnosis. This fact is because the hypnotist may make suggestions, but the assessment and perception of these suggestions in the subject's own mind that heralds the performance. The hypnotist is merely a vehicle that assists the issue in a trance, but it is the subject that processes the knowledge. The outcome is the same, however.

Self-hypnosis can be used in a somewhat similar manner to hypnotherapy and effectively resolve psychological difficulties, phobias, depression, and addictions. It is also used simply to facilitate a state of deep relaxation.

NLP

Any of you may have heard of NLP or (neurolinguistic programming). It originates from psychological counseling, coping with psychological problems, phobias, depression, behaviors, and learning disorders. The NLP approach is still commonly used but is now most widely used as a self-help tool to encourage well-being. This technique has seen a dramatic rise in popularity and is being used by clinicians for patients, business practitioners, life coaches, and self-help courses.

NLP hypnosis is used to treat psychological or behavioral disorders or simply to enhance one's sense of well-being. It's a perfect tool for inspiration and self-confidence.

Ericsonian Hypnosis

This form of hypnosis has several different names, covert hypnosis, covert hypnosis, black ops hypnosis, instant hypnosis, conversational hypnosis, but to mention a few. This method uses natural communication and encourages hypnotic induction without the participant being aware that this is happening.

Ericksonian hypnosis or conversational hypnosis was initiated by hypnotherapist Dr. Milton H. Erickson. After becoming ill with polio, Erickson perfected the use of words, holding him in bed for several years. During this time, he mastered using natural conversation to trigger hypnotic states without the subject's awareness.

This method of hypnosis can be used for those who are skeptical about hypnotherapy or more conventional hypnosis and is said to be more beneficial for those who are more skeptical about it.

This method can be used by those who are suspicious about hypnosis or unaware that they are being hypnotized. Skeptical subjects tend to be more sensitive to this technique. The use of hypnotic language and hypnosis methods in ordinary conversations can trigger trance very quickly. This trance state is low but very powerful.

This hypnosis approach was initially introduced as a hypnotherapy technique, but it has become more prevalent in everyday life. The method helps individuals to take greater control of their lives and to use these methods to support them in certain daily circumstances. There are several different courses available to teach these methods, saying that you can take care of others. This way is valid to some degree, and it is clear that this type of hypnosis is real and successful. The process is relatively simple, but it will take some time to learn the system.

What is Weight Loss Hypnosis?

In a super-sized country, people have many chances to eat and drink WAY too much, but what's behind obesity is typically more than a wish for a large number of fries. In America, the big dietary industry has evolved around obesity, pushing overweight people to pay a high price for trendy diets, drugs, or costly, high-risk surgeries. Through removing carbs or fat, taking medications or injections, sprinkling crystals on the food, using surgery, or consuming miracle diet potions, many dietitians momentarily lose their pounds-but do not lose the mind that leads to weight gain. The consequence is that, after all the hard work and potentially costing thousands of dollars, most dietitians get their weight back and become even more discouraged.

Weight loss hypnosis will help you improve the way you feel and manage your poor eating habits.

Weight Loss Hypnosis Breaks Down WHY You Eat

Hypnosis therapy has helped people lose weight sustainably by modifying their eating habits, reducing stress and pressure, and learning how to relax. Overeating has nothing to do with appetite but has more to do with high stress, racing thoughts, and other negative emotional feelings that food causes a person to be distracted from feeling.

Like all hypnosis, weight loss hypnosis uses the power of suggestion when people are in a relaxed state as long as the directions are compatible with what the individual needs to do first. Part of the emphasis is on changing tastes and decisions to healthier food choices and resolving the food cravings. Because many dieters have poor thinking habits that allow them to use donuts and cheesy bacon bowls to alter how they feel, weight loss hypnosis often helps you see yourself as an influential person who doesn't need food to improve something. You learn to see changing eating habits not as deprivation, but as empowering and simple because that's what you want to do first.

Does Weight Loss Hypnosis Work?

Hypnosis can be thought of as a skill-a technique that people use to relax, improve their attitude, and feel in a better, more optimistic, and more useful way. All hypnosis is "self-hypnosis," so the individual is 100 % responsible for how it works and what the effects are. The hypnotist is like a mentor who teaches and guides a person calmly and simply learns what they need to be successful. This way is all, of course, dependent on the DECISION that the person makes to lose weight in the first place-hypnosis is never a substitute for a personal decision. Neither the hypnotist nor the hypnosis itself can make a person do something. The person needs to want to lose weight so that hypnosis will help the decision, and sometimes they don't have to go on another diet again.

Why Hypnosis Is A Great Weight Loss Approach

Significant weight loss depends on your encouragement. When people start eating, they tend to be shot when they start. They may lose weight, but if progress slows down, they may be discouraged. And someone who has lost a considerable amount of weight plateaus at some stages as the body battles against weight loss.

When you work hard to lose, and you don't lose much, discouragement makes it easier to rationalize dropping off the wagon. You think, "I don't lose anyway, so I might as well have that hot fudge sundae." Or, "I didn't work out today, so just forget-the week is ruined." Weight loss hypnosis trains you to think like thin people, to make choices about food like these people, and to eat like thin people. Contrary to other thought, inherently slim people are not that way, since they still eat chicken and salad without dressing. Instead, they know what will feel good in their stomachs before they eat, so they know what needs in moderation. Then they understand when to avoid eating based on how they think and see treats as occasional little indulgences, not the constant need for unhealthy food that they later feel mentally and physically crappy about eating.

Hypnosis for weight loss encourages a healthy weight loss. It keeps your outlook lively, even when weight loss is sluggish at times. While weight loss will still fluctuate a little from week to week, the other outcomes of hypnosis, such as increased self-esteem, relaxation, inspiration, and a relaxed state of mind, continue to grow. Hypnosis shifts the link between food and feelings as it recreates the right state of mind in the direction of feeding. Since the procedure does not depend on medications and there are no diets of any sort, hypnosis is a gentle solution to weight loss that will make you slimmer, more comfortable, and with noticeable improvements in how you view food and your emotions.

As with all hypnosis, most people can respond to suggestions made when they are in a very relaxed state. A successful hypnotist will determine whether you are the right candidate for weight loss hypnosis based on the strength of your motivation to improve and your ability to take training and obey instructions.

How Do You Select A Weight-Loss Hypnotist?

Weight loss hypnosis is most effective when conducted by practitioners who have a lot of experience with hypnosis in general and weight loss hypnosis in particular. Make sure you inquire about their experience and their history of achievements working with many people losing weight. They should be able to display a lot of good results and to make real feedback and outcomes available to the public.

If you're ready to stop dieting forever and build a safe, easy attitude towards food, weight loss hypnosis might be right for you.

In recent years, weight loss hypnosis has created waves in the multi-million-dollar weight loss industry, selling itself as an innovative way to help people lose weight and keep their excess pounds off. These initiatives have moved people from famous movie stars to ordinary homemakers using weight loss hypnosis methods to help them lose weight and maintain their figures. With all recent trends in weight loss, is weight loss with hypnosis and over-hyped myth that doesn't work as advertised, or is it a miracle that people have been waiting for?

No matter what the ads display about how new weight loss hypnosis is, the fact is, these techniques have been in operation for many years. These same methods that are taught in weight loss hypnosis programs are also used to address other conditions in individuals such as smoking, pain management, anxiety disorders, and, of course, weight loss. Techniques used in weight loss hypnosis by many trained weight loss hypnosis practitioners are derived from existing and validated hypnosis techniques such as anchoring and association.

For several people, the term hypnosis often creates photos of people performing dumb antics under the direction of a stage hypnotist. As a result of this hypnosis depiction, people have been slow to take up hypnosis for weight loss methods or to approach a trained weight loss hypnosis practitioner for their weight control goals. While the stage hypnotic uses some of the ways of hypnosis, a proper weight loss hypnosis program is different from a variety of television hypnosis programs.

During a weight loss hypnosis program, a trained weight loss hypnosis practitioner can first consider what your expectations are for yourself. He or she will go over with you what is the present situation that you are in, what are the diet and eating habits that you have now, and where you want to be when the program is done. This stage is very critical because it sets the goals you commit to, and, indeed, you can achieve. This fact is important because, contrary to common belief, hypnosis can't work until deep down, you don't believe you can do it, or you don't want to do it. By carrying out a weight loss target that you're happy with, you're subconsciously more committed to the goal. The next step will be to get you to a profoundly relaxed state. It is in this condition that the hypnotherapist gives you ideas for healthy food choices and motivating words to help you lose weight. These ideas are aimed at your subconscious mind. Why to the mind of the subconscious? Your subconscious mind is a dominant part of your brain. It regulates your thoughts, your emotions, your attitudes, and your habits. By adding these ideas to your subconscious mind, your habits and feelings for food and exercise change. Many people have indicated that after hypnosis for weight loss services, they don't eat as much as they did before because they feel fuller and quicker after a small meal.

In addition to presenting you with ideas that encourage healthy nutrition and exercise, a trained weight loss hypnosis practitioner can also include you in setting up a plan for yourself. Goal-setting strategies will teach you exactly what to do, how to accomplish your goals, and how to evaluate your results. Seeing success during your weight loss hypnosis program will shape a positive feedback loop and motivate you to remain on track to meet the weight loss goals you set yourself.

Thus, weight loss hypnosis is real and is now helping people from all walks of life achieve their weight loss goals and give them back control of their lives by giving them a simple and easy way to achieve their desired level of health.

How to Use Hypnosis to Achieve Your Goals

Hypnosis has become a technique useful in the area of medicine and psychology. It has been used to relieve pain, resolve trauma, resolve addiction, and has been used by expectant mothers to make childbirth an enjoyable experience.

Apart from its various applications in medicine and psychology, hypnosis has also been used to help multiple achieve their goals. In reality, it's one of the strategies and tips for success that many people are now after breaking bad habits, improving self-confidence, and working toward your goals.

Practice helps you to go into deep relaxation, where you can give constructive feedback to your subconscious that allows you to shift negative thinking, bad habits, and other self-limiting thoughts that discourage you from achieving your goals. By the constructive feedback that you give to your subconscious during the trance state, you are re-training your mind to be productive and conquer the thoughts that contribute to your loss of self-confidence and self-esteem.

For example, if one of your personal goals were to lose weight, and you didn't seem to have the drive to keep up with it, you would need a little boost from your subconscious. Often our conscious mind can jump to getting negative thoughts about being hungry, being too exhausted to exercise, and worrying about putting it off, or worrying that you will never reach your goals or that you will fail. With a little support from your subconscious, you can get rid of those feelings that are putting you down right before you try to achieve your goals.

While you may have some professional hypnotherapists doing hypnosis for you, you may learn to do self-hypnosis where you can go through hypnosis without the help of the therapist.

Usually, this includes writing down constructive ideas that you can give to your subconscious, and then putting yourself in a state of deep relaxation by closing your eyes and taking your mind to a calm and quiet position to see yourself achieving your goals.

While hypnosis can significantly affect the transformation of these negative thoughts into positive ones, it does not take place overnight. Daily practice is required and, of course, recognize that individuals can undergo various levels of hypnosis, so it is necessary to continue the procedure until you get the desired results. You will also find hypnosis audios that can help you relax profoundly.

Indeed, if you're searching for tips on success or ways to help you accomplish your goals or change the thinking that keeps you from achieving what you want in life, you may find the answer in hypnosis.

CHAPTER TWO

SELF-HYPNOSIS

There have been so many debates lately about self-hypnosis. Let's talk about what self-hypnosis is before we get into what it can and can't do for us.

If you've ever been to a hypnotherapist, you might have been told that all hypnosis is self-hypnosis. Essentially, this is valid. What this signifies is that no one can make you go to hypnosis without your permission or cooperation. The media and stage hypnotists have led many of us to assume that hypnosis is an abnormal condition placed on us by those with mind control powers.

Nothing could have been further from these facts. Hypnosis is a natural state of mind that we all undergo many times a day. Whenever your mind is so concentrated that you don't know what's going on around you, you're in a hypnotic state. We are in a state of hypnosis, also watching TV or reading or playing if we fall out of the moment and into our minds and where our attention is concentrated.

There are other times when we get into a light hypnotic state. For example, when we're called to the office, we're in a highly suggestive state. When we're in a big crowd at a concert or other event, we're in a mild form of hypnosis. These are only a few examples of when we're in hypnosis in our everyday daily lives.

So, we may gather that hypnosis is a state of mind where we're concentrating on everything other than what's going on right in front of us. Or we're so focused on what's going on in front of us that we lose consciousness to anything else. It is a condition where we can suggest that we can internalize knowledge and make it part of our fact or belief system. An example of this is when we watch a movie and weep at the end of it. Even if the events didn't happen to us, we're so involved that we can feel the feelings as if they were happening to us.

Of course, when we talk about self-hypnosis in a clinical context, we're not talking about these experiences. We are talking about a deliberate phase in which we take our attention away from our immediate surroundings and place ourselves in a modified state of mind for a particular reason.

So How Do We Do Self-Hypnosis?

There are several ways to do self-hypnosis as there are people, but for this writing, I'm going to explain an easy but successful method that everyone can do.

The first thing you want to do is find a quiet spot where you won't be interrupted. Only allow yourself a decent half-hour. Switch off your phone and ask the kids to be calm and have fun this time. However, in an emergency, realize that you can quickly be stimulated and return to ordinary awakening consciousness, without difficulty.

Get cozy, whether you're sitting or lying down. If you like, you can have soft music in the background. Many meditative music recordings are suitable for self-hypnosis. Some people are using theme to take them further into relaxation.

Now, just concentrate on your breathing. See your breath come in and out of your nose. Feel the air coming into your body. See your stomach rise and fall. Often breathing exercise is followed by the concept of "breathe in relaxation and calmness and breathe our tension and stress."

You may also use relaxation to get you to a peaceful state of deep peace and quiet. Imagine the muscles around your eyes begin to relax and get limp. Then take the feeling to the top of your head. Feel all the muscles in your head, face, and neck, let go and relax. Use this strategy to go all the way down your body, relax, and soothe down.

Using terms like "deeper and deeper into relaxation," "going all the way down," "calm relaxed relaxation," etc. in your mind as you breathe and feel all the tension flowing out of your muscles.

Counting backward is another excellent way to get further into relaxation. "Ten going down ... 9 twice as comfortable as before ... 8 still going down ... etc."

You can begin to experience a physical sensation like floating or tingling or numbness. You may note a temperature change, either warming or cooling down. Each has a unique experience with hypnosis. Pay attention to the senses and see how you're going to perceive hypnosis.

At this point, a lot of people would wonder, "What is the difference between self-hypnosis and meditation?"

Meditation is a method to clear the mind. Hypnosis is similar in that you may relax and monitor your breathing, but that's where the similarities end. Hypnosis has a specific function attached to it. Rather than being transparent, the mind is primarily involved, but in a way that is different from the normal state of consciousness.

You're going to go into hypnosis with a purpose. If the reason you use hypnosis is for stress relief, for example, you may want to keep me calm and comfortable all day. I feel the tension slipping out of my fingers and toes. "You can repeat this many times and perceive or picture the pressure escaping your body through your fingers and toes. It might seem like static electricity, or you may see angry gnomes marching out of the ends of your feet.

Imagination plays a significant role in hypnosis. Visualizing or imagining the result you desire helps introduce the idea into your subconscious mind. Once the concept is in your subconscious mind, it becomes part of your daily life.

The subconscious mind does not know the difference between truth and imagination when you envision or imagine something that your subconscious mind will bring into your life. When you go into self-hypnosis with a particular goal in mind and repeat the intention, it becomes part of you.

You will find that when you are in hypnosis, you have a boss. This way is a part of your mind that stays in charge at all times. This area is the part of your mind that will reiterate the intent. It will also get you out of hypnosis at the agreed time.

To come out of hypnosis, say to yourself, "I'm going to count from one to five and counting five, I'm going to open my eyes and go back to regular awakening consciousness." Now, count ... "One, coming up slowly ... two, feeling refreshed and rested and energetic ... three, feeling my body back in the bed ... four, remembering all the helpful stuff I've said to my subconscious mind today..., five, eyes open up.

Self-hypnosis will enable us to do a lot of good. You can lower the blood pressure if you choose to. You can alleviate stress or change sleep patterns. You can enhance your study habits. There are several things you can do with self-hypnosis, but there is the one really significant thing you can't do with self-hypnosis, and that is counseling.

The distinction between the hypnotist and the hypnotherapist is counseling. The hypnotherapist uses psychological techniques when the person is in a state of hypnosis to create changes in their life. Hypnotherapy is a partnership between the hypnotherapist and the person. It is not possible for those in hypnosis to ask questions and search deeper and use the techniques required to locate the source of the issue.

Self-hypnosis is very helpful for the reduction of stress and other related problems. It is essential to have a hypnotherapist working with a clinical background to get to the root of the problem and find solutions.

While you're searching for a hypnotherapist, find somebody you're related to that you feel comfortable with. Ensure the therapist is qualified to do the job. If possible, check their credentials. Hypnotherapy is not governed by some government bodies so that anybody can hang a shingle and call themselves a hypnotherapist. Make sure the person you're working with is well educated and competent in their medical practice.

Ways to Use Self Hypnosis

Self-hypnosis is a known way of helping individuals to accomplish specific goals. It is known by the medical brotherhood and is not one of those 'alternative' methods that may or may not be real science. It is associated with the overcoming phobias, or as a way of soothing oneself during times of stress, and is very useful in coping with both.

However, it's only relatively recently that hypnotism has become known as a way of helping you achieve your business goals and helping you improve your attitude to life and eliminate the roadblocks to your ambitions. However, DIY hypnotism is still a mystery to most people, even though many online courses will teach you how to do it.

While this strategy will help you accomplish objectives, it must be precise, and it must be feasible. Taking the attainable first, you're going to get nowhere by hypnotizing yourself to pick the winning lottery numbers, because you have no power over what they are. Likewise, you cannot hypnotize yourself to keep your best girl from marrying your worst enemy: that again is beyond your reasonable control (though you may try!).

When using self-hypnosis to accomplish your goals, these goals must be attainable without supernatural intervention, but by your own constructive acts. In reality, most of the benefits of hypnosis can also be obtained if you can build a positive mindset without it. But that's easy to tell, but it's not that easy for most of us to do it.

For example, if you want to lose 3 pounds of weight per week, you could hypnotize yourself to accomplish that: or you could eat less and exercise more. However, self-hypnotism has a substantial part in achieving your goals. It would help if you had the self-confidence and motivation that is difficult to sustain when times are tough but can be obtained by hypnotizing yourself to keep going when others can give up.

One of the critical laws of self-hypnosis is that you have to be precise. You can't just say to yourself, "I want to be successful." You have to be very precise than that, and during your hypnotherapy or self-hypnosis session, say something more like, "I want to make that presentation a good one," or, "I want to boost my job performance," or, "I want to do well during this meeting."

Make practical wishes, hypnotize yourself to have the right mindset, and get your expertise and abilities out of your subconscious, and then you will succeed. Suddenly, no amount of hypnotism can get you named CEO or President. It's not magic; it's a way to give you the trust you need to achieve your goals. It's not the stage show of a hypnotist where he seems to make subjects do as he asks. Self-hypnosis is a well-known way to help you concentrate on what's important, help you relax, and help you make the most of your abilities.

So, given that self-hypnosis is a known tool for you to boost your concentration and focus on your goals, it should be clear to you that you need to accept specific goals that you want to accomplish. Are they realistic, huh? Are they for your benefit and also for the use of your employer or your business? Objectives that are either impractical or that do not help others in the same way they help you (and therefore do not receive their support) may be unattainable. No amount of hypnotism will allow you to accomplish goals such as these.

However, if these aims are practical and would also help most people if you could only accomplish them, using self-hypnosis to achieve your goals would seem reasonable, and your inner mind would agree with you. Then, and only then, will this technique work to allow you to achieve your goals.

The Self-hypnosis Abilities of Weight Loss

For decades, men have used hypnosis to treat several illnesses as well as psychological issues. Doctors and alternative medicine practitioners claim that hypnosis is an important therapeutic technique to correct specific problems. For example, smoking, which is a habit that is considered challenging to break, may be cured by hypnosis. By definition, all hypnosis is self-hypnosis since you are an active participant. It doesn't matter if you have someone else doing hypnosis, but it's always your mind that's the topic. And for hypnosis to be effective, you need your explicit, conscious consent. Hypnosis can also be performed with individuals who have trouble making their diet program work. Here are some essential Self Hypnosis Weight Loss Technique you can use to support your weight problem.

First of all, the Self-Hypnosis Method for Weight Loss is to be in a position where you can have peace and quiet. Ideally, you should be in a room where you could also be in a relaxed position. It is recommended that you wear loose clothing when doing this. If you like, you can listen to slow music so that you can relax, and your heart rate can be reduced to 60 beats per second. Your muscles need to be fully relaxed, and your mind clear from any thoughts. You must not be within reach for any distraction to do this. You should leave your cell phone behind, too.

When you have achieved complete relaxation and liberated your mind from all emotions, the Second Self Hypnosis Weight Loss Technique will visualize you releasing yourself from your body. Daydreaming is a type of self-hypnosis, so you have an idea of how to do it. To be successful, order your body and mind to achieve the weight loss program you desired. Hypnosis is very efficient in changing a person's mind following hypnosis. You can do this repeatedly when you say a mantra in a long, repetitive, and meditative way. When you become conscious, you will now have the drive to practice the weight loss program you've always wanted.

CHAPTER THREE

THE BENEFITS OF HYPNOSIS

Hypnosis has become useful when people are surrounded by too much tension in their jobs, and their daily lives are in a rat race. In reality, many people are searching for alternative ways to de-stress and eliminate the many negatives in their lives.

Aside from these stressors in life, several factors prevent a person from being what he wants to be and allowing him to achieve his goals. Among these are anxiety and anxieties and negative feelings that have been hidden deep inside the subconscious.

One of the methods most people have used these days is hypnosis, and, in reality, it has also been commonly used in the medical industry as a treatment for psychotherapy. If you're interested in learning more about hypnosis, here are some of the top advantages of hypnosis.

1. Help with phobias and fears. Hypnotherapy has also been effective in resolving deep-rooted fears and phobias that are impossible to conquer consciously. If you don't want to be forced to confront your fears, then hypnosis can be your way to beat it.

2. It helps you to regulate your weight. If you find it very difficult to control your diet and weight, and you lack the motivation to do so, you can find hypnosis as a helpful solution to helping you maintain your weight loss issues. Most of the time, weight loss attempts fail due to a lack of motivation or control over their emotions. If you want to

support when it comes to losing weight or trying to keep fit, you can also take advantage of the benefits of hypnosis in this field.

3. Overcoming dependency. Another essential application and advantage of hypnosis are helping you conquer addiction and other bad behaviors that are difficult to control consciously. Alcoholic or opioid abuse are the two most common things that are impossible to manage actively. If you think you're having trouble controlling your addictions, hypnosis will help make the process smoother.

4. Getting rid of the habit of smoking. Yeah, stopping smoking can be very difficult, especially if you've been in the practice for a long time, especially if you're a chain smoker. If you desire to seek help from your subconscious to reduce the temptations of cigarette lighting, hypnosis can be helpful.

5. Enhancing memory recollection. Memory retrieval is another of the many applications and advantages of hypnosis. This way is also a good use of hypnosis in the courts and in items that require some recall.

Apart from all these applications and advantages of hypnosis, you can also render hypnosis a good tool to boost your ability to manipulate and convince people. Of course, it is vital that you positively use hypnosis and not hurt anyone. You can also find this useful and helpful, particularly if you're in the sales industry.

Things You Should Know About Hypnosis

Are you considering hypnosis to help you fight a specific life? Good for you, man! Hypnosis is an effective technique to help people solve the issues in their lives. It is successful over and over in studies and has been endorsed by the American Medical Association, the American Psychiatric Association, and the American Psychological Association for decades.

However, there are some things you need to know about hypnosis before you plunge into the process. Understanding these items ahead of time will help you make the most of whatever work you can do with hypnosis.

(1) Hypnosis is a condition of focus and relaxation. Many people have seen hypnosis used in several stage shows, and as a result, they have a somewhat warped understanding of what it is. It's always believed that a hypnotist will manipulate you or make you do dumb or humiliating stuff, but that's simply not true. An individual undergoing hypnosis is still in charge and will not do something morally or ethically unacceptable

to them. Hypnosis is a state of absorption, focus, and concentration that makes it easier for us to consider and act on selective, appropriate ideas and suggestions.

(2) You will be able to undergo hypnosis if you want to. Since hypnosis is a state of focus and concentration, if you can do a relatively good job of focusing, you will experience a state of hypnosis. There appear to be several "hypnotizables," with certain people able to go deeply into hypnotic states and show predictable hypnotic phenomena, and others who have a hard time doing so. People in the latter group seem to be extremely critical thinkers, but they may also undergo the condition of hypnosis. People of this bent are typically very good at concentration, so with a specialist used to dealing with a wide variety of individuals, even highly analytical, logical thinkers will undergo hypnosis.

(3) Many people undergo hypnotic environments every day. If you understand the concept of hypnosis as mentioned above, it should be noted that most people experience hypnosis very frequently, maybe even several times a day, and they do! Any examples: a child who gets so focused on his game system that he doesn't hear his mom calling him for dinner. Or the partner who is so interested in her computer work that an hour passes, and she feels it's only been 15 minutes. Or maybe you, when you made the usual drive home from work, and when you

pulled into the driveway, couldn't remember the specifics of the drive (this is called "highway hypnosis"). The hypnotist can simply make the process clear and guided for the intent of the improvement that you are seeking.

(4) You can recall what's going on in your hypnosis session. Many people are afraid that they will be in some altered state of consciousness that will not allow them to recognize what's going on during hypnosis, but that's not true. You will recall, be conscious, and be in charge of the entire process.

(5) Hypnosis is not a magic bullet. Hypnosis is a fantastic way to overcome anxiety, panic, fears, phobias, frustration, depression, or help people lose weight, handle stress better, or develop self-esteem and trust. But you need to be an enthusiastic and willing participant! There are several problems where hypnosis is more of an addition to other work that a person does-such as weight loss, so hypnosis would be more effective if you already have a diet and exercise plan in place. It also requires good communication between you and the professional with whom you work, so be ready to share with him or her what your issues are, what your ambitions are, and any questions you might have along the way.

Treatment of Stress with Self-hypnosis

Why does anyone want to practice self-hypnosis and learn how to do that? One explanation for this is helping to minimize pain. Getting pain in one's life can be consuming even though it's not persistent. Pain can hurt as well as trigger stress. The problem even takes away the quality of life of a person, whether it's a daily event or every few months, which needs to be monitored.

Different people have different causes for their suffering from a disease to injury. It can be handled with medication occasionally. However, this drug can't work for everybody, or you may prefer to treat the pain without medication. One way to do this is to increase the popularity of self-hypnosis. This technique is thought to put a stop to the discomfort.

Well, if you haven't seen a doctor for the pain, it may be a good idea to get started. This way is to make sure there's nothing serious about the problem that the doctor wants to handle. It's also going to help you know the root of the pain. Now, you can focus on that painful spot. The use of self-hypnosis only treats pain, not the real cause. You will still feel better and struggle less. It may also be used by others to work with their medications.

Self-hypnosis also works instantly, and an important note of pain relief can be seen when used regularly. It is recommended that this procedure be implemented at the beginning of each day. There are ways to learn about self-hypnosis from books to experts. Knowing how to do self-hypnosis correctly ensures that there is a greater chance of it working. When someone knows the process and tries it over and over again, it's going to be simpler. It's all down to what you think is going to work for you. You can try self-hypnosis, whether you like it or not.

Some individuals pursue self-hypnosis and give it a shot, but find it doesn't work for them. They're choosing to try something else. Others take self-hypnosis to help relieve pain. They discover that they like it, and it works for them. They learned the right technique, and they were able to bring it into their everyday routine. Many feel it won't hurt to try self-hypnosis, particularly if they're in such pain, they think they don't have a choice, and nothing else helps.

Also, self-hypnosis helps relieve stress and is one of the techniques used to relieve stress at home and in the corporate world.

After Self Hypnosis

If you practice self-hypnosis regularly and want to get the most out of your time, it might be helpful to note some principles for enjoying successful self-hypnosis sessions, such as:-

1) Practice Increases Productivity and Capacity

Much like every other discipline or skill, daily practice helps to improve and enhance your skills. You will learn a lot and experience positive improvements and a sense of peace right from your first session. Continue practicing your self-hypnosis, and you will have a habit of calming stress and tension.

2) Self-hypnosis is not a competition

Efficient and long-lasting relaxation is not about rhythm or volume. Be patient and take your time, and eventually, even before you planned, you will be relaxed and peaceful, and have a sense of inner peace.

3) Regular practice

If you do something half-heartedly, you're likely to end up with a half-hearted outcome. Commit yourself to the practice of self-hypnosis every day. Positive results are going to inspire you to proceed.

4) Where is it to be done?

You may perform self-hypnosis in a variety of different locations. And some people feel secure enough to do that on tubes and busses. Any of the office employees take time off during their lunch break. When you're new to this relaxing phase, it may be better to choose the comfort and security of your home.

5) Be Fussy-Be happy with me.

Although you can enjoy relaxing in any spot, as described above, you can enhance your relaxation by being furious about your surroundings. This way will involve asking that no other person in your home interferes with your set self-hypnosis time and that possible noises, such as phones, are shut off, and all other distractions are controlled.

6) Settle yourself to calmness

Check that your posture is relaxed and that your back and head are well supported. Your body is going to lose heat, so make sure you're warm enough. The more confident you are in your ease, the better and the more profound relaxation you can feel.

7) The approval of

You will find that one session of self-hypnosis is very deep and intense, and the next one feels lighter. This section is all right, and it's a natural part of the process. Only acknowledge that this is going to happen, and you're going to get right out of it.

8) Cluttered Mind — Clear Mind

Occasionally, your mind may seem still, and your thoughts are few and far between. You're going to dream a day and enjoy this state of respect. You'll even have moments when the mind is cluttered and over-active. These are natural interactions, and once again, the best way is to embrace what you get at that moment.

9) It's all right to have a fixed time in mind

It might be wise to have a defined time before beginning your self-hypnosis. You are much more likely to wake up and then get on with the rest of the day. If you don't set a time, you can find that you're going to sleep. This way is perfect if it's your bedtime, but it's not that good if you have other things to do after your workout. Have a watch or clock that you might momentarily open your eyes to see if you need to see how many minutes have passed since you began. After a while, the internal clock would be strong enough to measure more precisely how many minutes have passed.

10) Flexible self-hypnosis pacing

It's a good idea, initially, to make the length of the self-hypnosis the same, e.g., 20 minutes. After a while, you can vary the size to be longer or shorter, depending on your circumstances or needs.

CHAPTER FOUR

THE POWER OF GUIDED MEDITATION

Guided meditation (sometimes referred to as guided imaging meditation) is literally "meditation with the aid of a guide." It's one of the best ways to get into a state of deep relaxation and inner stillness, and it's one of the most effective ways to reduce tension and bring about meaningful personal change.

What's it like?

Guided meditation is usually experienced with the aid of a meditation teacher or by listening to a recording.

Your meditation guide will ask you to sit down comfortably, or you might be asked to lie down in some situations. You then listen to your guide as they guide you through a series of soothing visualizations. When you slowly relax and become more and more still, tension falls away, and your mind becomes clearer and more transparent.

When you are in this profoundly relaxed state of mind, your subconscious is open to constructive feedback, and your guide will use this opportunity to take you on an inner journey designed to change one or more aspects of your life. For example, guided meditation might be geared to personal empowerment and positive thinking. Another can focus on emotional healing or spiritual growth. You may be taken on a guided journey to unlock your full potential, or you may choose to go on a guided trip only for the pure enjoyment of deep relaxation.

As you can see now, guided meditation can be an experience that is not only calming, but one that strengthens your sense of self, that changes your outlook in positive ways, and that encourages you to live your life to the fullest.

It's an effortless and enjoyable experience that results in deep relaxation, stress removal, and heightened enjoyment of life.

At the end of your meditation, your guide will gradually bring you back to a state of ordinary consciousness, making you feel refreshed, rejuvenated, and comfortable. Driven meditation can be as short as 5 minutes or as long as an hour, depending on your personal preference. In most cases, guided meditation of 20 minutes or longer is recommended if you want to achieve a genuinely deep state of relaxation and optimize positive benefits.

What makes guided meditation different from that?

Most conventional meditation methods enable you to take charge of your own consciousness by focusing on a single focal point. This point of emphasis may be your breathing, and it may be a physical movement, or, more generally, it may be a mantra-a sound, an expression, or a phrase that you mentally repeat to yourself.

While these effective meditation techniques are perfect for creating inner stillness and improving the ability to focus, some people find it challenging to master.

One of the critical reasons why guided meditation is such a common alternative to conventional meditation methods is that it does not require any prior preparation or effort to enjoy it. Even if you are someone who finds it incredibly difficult to let go of your emotions, even if you are positively overwhelmed or overloaded with mental activity. So you can easily attain inner stillness and peace of mind when you are properly guided to do so.

Since this kind of meditation is so simple, it is beneficial for people who are new to meditation. Guided meditation, however, may also be of great benefit to people who are very experienced in meditation. Experienced meditators also use directed imaging meditations to undergo deeper or more vivid meditation, to dig deeper into their minds than they would usually be able to do, or to target a particular area of personal growth that they would like to discuss.

Guided meditation also differs from conventional meditation in that it uses music and nature sounds to enhance the meditation experience.

The role of music and other nature sounds in the guided meditation of images

Directed imaging recordings typically include peaceful meditation music that helps you relax as you're led by meditation. Think about how much of the difference a good soundtrack makes to a movie, and guided meditation benefits from music in a similar way. Music adds another layer of speech and complexity to your guided journey of meditation while calming your mind.

It's also not rare for guided meditation CDs and MP3s to contain the sounds of nature. These sounds are very calming, and they can also be used to increase the vividness of the visualizations you encounter during your meditation. For example, if you are directed to imagine yourself standing on a sandy beach, then your experience of visualization would be more authentic if you can hear the sound of ocean waves.

In contrast to conventional meditation, where the purpose is to achieve mental silence through focus exercises, guided imaging meditations rely on a vibrant tapestry of visualizations, music, and ambient sounds to relax, captivate the attention and immerse you in an inner journey. Since this inner path can be customized to achieve particular results, guided meditation can be far more critical than conventional passive meditation methods for making positive personal changes in your life.

Using Guided Meditations is the best way for you to start a meditation practice or to continue daily meditation practice. Guided meditations come in various formats, audio, and video, and are intended to support you with a wide range of issues. You can find guided meditation in any subject, ranging from dwindling anxiety to cosmic energy meditation.

Top 3 Benefits of Guided Meditation

1. Better Attention-People who have already learned how to meditate and use guided meditation can keep their focus on the task at hand. They will relax and face the rest of their day with a concentrated being. Driven meditation walks you through focusing on the object of meditation, which forces the mind to concentrate on the purpose, not the distractions that usually occur. Use guided meditation for five to ten minutes a day; the mind gets a break from all the tension it's been under. It leaves you with a sense of calm.

2. Energy Increase-As soon as you have completed your guided meditation; you should be comfortable and refreshed. You'll feel like you can face the rest of the day with certainty and look past the root of stress to find a healthy, consistent solution. If you have reached the level of consciousness you provide guided meditation, you will be able to do more and do what is required for others and yourself. You will need to practice the mind from the ordinary, distracted mind to the concentrating mind, and then to the meditating mind. It takes time to work your way through these three stages, but once you learn it, it's easier to get to the meditating mind.

3. Reduce Negative Thoughts-Guided meditation is a perfect way to get level-headed during the day and reduce the negative aspects of stress. It just takes a few minutes, and you're going to feel incredibly refreshed and revived. If you have a big meeting that makes you anxious, take time for a little guided meditation, and you'll be able to focus on the discussion. It can be used in other ways to restore your composure, and it can only be an asset to your life.

The way guided meditation works is for the practitioners to lie or sit in a comfortable position. When this happens, a story is told that takes you on a conscious journey while still subconsciously imagining the story. When this happens, the body will relax, and all the tension will melt away. The only knowledge you have is the words of the story, the tone of the voice, the background music, and any sound effects that accompany the recording or the spoken voice. This way will encourage you to go into deep relaxation. And if one falls asleep, the subconscious is still active, and therefore the advantages and effects of this meditation technique will still be achieved.

As you listen, you will be directed to various levels of concentration while profoundly calming your body. When the supervised session is finished, the practitioners are taken back to consciousness.

There are many advantages to this form of meditation. Like all meditations, they help relax and focus the body, assist in recovery, and help the body protect itself from further stress and stress. Also, other advantages shall include:

- Drop-in heart rate
- Stabile blood pressure
- Enhancement of self-confidence and self-esteem
- Clearness of mind
- Increased concentration and emphasis
- Feeling in control and at ease
- Happiness and optimism

As far as the sort of meditation you're looking for depends on what you're looking for. If you want to lose weight, there are several books and tapes available for guided weight loss meditation. If you're going to contact the afterlife to pursue higher spiritual guidance, you will find outlets for this as well. Only the fundamental problems of self-esteem and self-confidence have a place in a guided meditation and are generous support when you need some positive affirmations in your life.

No matter what problem you choose to deal with or what form of guided meditation you choose, always note that the choices you make are yours and no one else.

Guided Meditation for Weight Loss

If you are a compulsive eater, you might have encountered various food failures after traumatic events in your life. You may find it easy to stick to your diet initially, but inevitably the temptation to binge eating overwhelms you when stressful events happen in your life. Even if you manage to lose weight on your diet, you can find yourself quickly getting it all back. Because no one can foresee the future, and you can't put your life on hold to go on a diet; if you find like you're having difficulty sticking to a diet because of the temptation to eat compulsively. Then it's crucial to fix your problems so that you can lose weight comfortably and keep it off.

Guided meditation for compulsive eating allows you to eat more carefully. Mindful eating is the opposite of unconscious eating. Eating food when watching TV and paying little attention to the taste or texture of food, and eating food as soon as possible are two examples of mindless eating. This way can lead to overeating and binge eating, as when you're eating unintentionally, it's hard to recognize when you're full. You feel the urge to consume more food to enjoy eating, contributing to more calories every day.

Conversely, when you eat carefully, you pay attention to all the specifics of the food you eat-noting the taste and texture of each bite you take and slowing down the rate at which you eat. By taking the time to appreciate food in this way, you can feel more satisfied by eating a smaller amount of food. Eating more slowly makes your stomach know when it's full-sometimes it can take up to 20 minutes for your stomach to signal to your brain that it's full and you're no longer hungry. By consuming a smaller amount of food, you will consume fewer calories during the day, leading to a healthy and steady weight loss.

Loving your soul and body

Many individuals who have been hurt all their lives will never hear the words, "I'm sorry," from others who have hurt them. Those esteem people in your life who have harmed you without atoning for their actions make it more challenging to overcome. To recover the perspective of the facts, you need to inventory your relationship. Look at the conduct and the acts of others in these relationships in accordance with the values of fairness, integrity, and affection. Start to set the necessary boundaries for the people you encounter. After all, this is complete; you will find a path to your recovery that includes a significant individual. You are this guy! When you look at your life as an adult, you are the one person responsible for your decisions, including the choices you make about relationships. You must rely on your unique talents and talents to see reality and discover the true meaning of life. A holistic approach to body and mind relations will encourage a higher degree of awareness that can overcome the chaos of your life.

Without creating a solid body and mind, I believe that you will continue to be vulnerable to the irrationality of those caught up in turmoil. I think that many people out there who have suffered best with the pressures of family, jobs, and relationship issues have shown the potential to obtain a positive perspective of life through physical and spiritual practice. These practices enabled many people to stay grounded in reality and helped them to realize what is real happiness and goodness in life. Exercise instantly takes people to the here and now. You begin to notice that the parts of the body are being exerted and begin to refocus your attention on the body. This way could sound minor and not worth the time and effort. Once you become more consistent with your workout routine, you will begin to experience the euphoria you will gain from your workout. During these periods, you will reach a higher level of consciousness if you allow yourself to lose the emotional balance that you have become so used to maintaining. In years of hurt and violence, many people tend to lose themselves mentally, emotionally, and sexually. They look at themselves as evil, hideous people, and sometimes equate their physical and emotional selves with their bad feelings. That's why I think you need to restore a good picture of yourself. I believe that you can do this by cultivating your body and soul.

Holistic Approach:

A holistic approach to wellness includes taking care of the mind, body, and soul. It's not all about physical fitness anymore; it's got to be the whole package deal! It makes much sense to take care of every single essential faculty of your being, because face it, how can you be genuinely safe if you're a psychological and emotional mess under that ideal six-dimensional body?

Here are the top five tips to get you started on the journey to holistic self-development and satisfaction:

1. Eat well. Self-development begins with a healthy constitution, which means maintaining a well-balanced diet. Nourish your body, mind, and soul with foods that come from fresh, chemical-free ingredients such as organic greens, hormone-free dairy products, and whole grains. Vitamins and minerals that you extract from such foods keep your body's functions in check, make you less resistant to illnesses. Such as common cold, help stave off depression and give you the overall glow that no beauty product will ever equal. Live right, live well, and eat with moderation.

2. Say goodbye to severe chemicals. If you're still using really strong chemicals to clean your home, let's say, trash them now! Not only can they affect the environment, but they also expose you to contaminants that can affect your health. If you've ever washed your bathroom with industrial-strength bleach, then you know how the perfume alone will make you

dizzy and make you irritable afterward. The invisible consequences, on the other hand, are what it can do to your lungs; bleaching chemicals can burn your lungs and leave lasting marks in you. Get rid of all toxic chemicals in your cupboard and stick to natural sources to preserve your mind, body, and soul.

3. Meditate on that. Meditation is perfect for self-development because it helps you interact with yourself far from the madness of the daily world. It also nurtures your mind, body, and soul in one go with its "all-in-one bundle" of healthy breathing, resting mentally and physically, and curing any emotional pains and pains you have. Try to integrate meditation time at least three times a week to rejuvenate yourself more if you happen to be working in a fast-paced, high-pressure job. Find a particular spot in your house where you can meditate in silence for at least half an hour and make sure you tell the people who live with you not to bother you unless there is anything highly urgent. This period is the time you need for yourself.

4. Spend time with your loved ones. Nothing soothes your mind, body, and soul like being in the company of people who mean the world to you! Significant others, children, parents, and our dearest friends unfailingly bring us so much joy even in the darkest hour. So, on the days where you feel you might

use your loved ones to pick me up, schedule quality time with them, and use that opportunity to reconnect, reflect and reassess what matters in your life. And if you feel motivated to broaden your inner circle, meet and mingle with other like-minded people. Building your support network is always a marvel of self-development as the more people you have in your life, the more positive and comfortable you feel.

5. Indulge yourself in an occasional massage. Anyone would have been hard-pressed to turn a massage down! It's one of the best ways to rejuvenate your mind, body, and soul, especially after a stressful week in your office. A calm environment, a sensation of loving hands kneading your body like dough, a calming fragrance of candles and oils are a formula for guaranteed relaxation. If you can't afford a professional masseuse, your partner may be able to step up to the challenge! Get a massage at least once in a month, and maybe a little more often, if the essence of your work is more physically and emotionally exhausting than most workers. The occasional indulgence is perfect for self-development as you come out to feel a much happier person after each session.

Increase your Self-Esteem Easily

Self-esteem is a mixture of self-esteem, self-esteem, self-respect, and self-integrity. It's a psychological term used to explain how a person feels about himself or herself. High self-esteem implies a high value put on the self, while low self-esteem suggests the opposite.

Abraham Maslow claims that psychological wellbeing is based on the heart and that it is possible only when the heart of a person is fundamentally embraced, cherished, and valued by others and by himself or herself. According to Jack Canfield, "Self-esteem is based on feeling capable and feeling lovable."

Self-esteem and self-image are interlinked. The word self-image is used to define a person's mental image of himself. Self-image is contributing to self-esteem. During early childhood, we create mental representations of ourselves: who we are, what we are good at, how we look, and what our strengths and weaknesses may be. Our memories and our interactions with other people will make these mental images clearer inside of us. Over time, these mental self-images will build our sense of self-esteem. Self-esteem is about emotions that we create within ourselves as a result of external influences. Self-esteem is how much we feel welcomed, respected, and appreciated by others, and how much we embrace, love, and respect ourselves. It's the combination of the two factors that form our self-esteem.

Usually, self-esteem is described in terms of how we view ourselves and our characteristics. According to Stanley Coppersmith, a groundbreaking researcher in the field, it is "personal assessment of worthiness that is reflected in the attitudes of the individual towards himself."

Strong self-esteem means that we are self-confident enough not to need the validation of others.

How is it developed?

Thoughts, relationships, and perceptions build self-esteem. Self-esteem starts to develop as early as adolescence, and factors that affect it include the likeness of one's own thoughts and beliefs, how others respond, experience at school, work and community, disability, illness, injury, culture, faith, and even one's position and place in society. Low self-esteem arises when a person does not see himself as possessing the qualities he admires. Unfortunately, people with low self-esteem typically have the attributes they respect, but they can't see it because they programmed their self-image that way. Dr. Michael Miller, editor-in-chief of the Harvard Mental Health Letter, says, "It is more likely that self-esteem will come from an accurate self-understanding, recognition of one's true talents, and satisfaction in supporting others." People who are closer to you, like parents, siblings, colleagues, teachers, and other interactions, and your relationship with these people will have a significant effect. Self-esteem is developed in your early childhood and matures in late adolescence. Whenever a person stabilizes his or her sense of being in charge of his or her own destiny, he or she starts to express self-esteem. Family relationship plays a vital role in deciding our self-esteem. It's how others treat us that show us if we're important. The feeling that we are cared for or worth it can form our level of self-esteem. This fact is related to the reception of approval from others. Yet, based on early life experiences and their social roles, women frequently seek acceptance more than men. By the age of sixteen, more girls than boys begin to report low self-esteem. According to Dove Research: The Real Truth About Beauty: 7 out of 10 girls feel that they're not good enough or that they don't measure up in any way, like their appearance, success at school, and relationships.

How important is self-esteem?

According to Brian Tracy, "Your self-esteem is probably the most important aspect of your personality. It precedes and predicts your success in almost everything you do. Your level of self-esteem is actually your level of mental health. To perform at your best and feel better about yourself, you should be in a constant state of self-esteem."

Self-esteem is vital to people as it gives them more courage to face life. Self-esteem would make it possible for a person to have more optimism and drive to achieve their goals. People with low self-esteem typically feel inadequate and may not perform well in various circumstances. They came up with false thoughts that no one would consider them or like them. On the other hand, people with positive self-esteem will feel good about their world and then feel good about themselves. They can do things more effectively, and by doing so, they can feel proud of their achievements and themselves.

Feeling good about ourselves will encourage us to enjoy life more and more. Feeling that we are welcomed, loved, and appreciated means that we have healthy self-esteem and that feeling will be mirrored in our relationships.

One of the biggest factors of broken relationships is low self-esteem.

Developing self-esteem helps us to be content with our lives. This way is the feeling that makes you believe that you deserve happiness. It is crucial to recognize this belief, the belief that you deserve to be happy and pleased. With this belief, you will treat others with dignity and goodwill, thereby preferring rich interpersonal relationships and avoiding negative ones. Possessing little to no self-respect can lead people to become unhappy, to fall short of their potential, or to accept abusive circumstances and relationships. Many studies have shown that low self-esteem leads to stress, depression, and anxiety. Research shows a strong relationship between high self-esteem and several positive outcomes, including satisfaction, modesty, resilience, and optimism. Self-esteem plays a part in almost everything that you do.

Can You Develop a Healthy Self Esteem?

The fact is, self-esteem is not entirely stable. A study released by the American Psychological Association found that self-esteem is the lowest among young adults, but rises during adulthood and peaks at 60 years of age, just before declining again. Researchers in the study assessed the self-esteem of 3,617 U.S. individuals. Women had, on average, lower self-esteem than men did much of their adulthood, but self-esteem converged as men and women reached their 80s and 90s. Blacks and whites had similar self-esteem levels in their early adulthood and middle age. The lead author of the report, Ulrich Orth, Ph.D., said: "Self-esteem is linked to improved health, less criminal activity, lower levels of depression and, overall, greater achievement in life. It is, therefore, important to learn more about how the average person's self-esteem changes over time."

Your thoughts are the greatest source of self-esteem, and these thoughts are beyond your influence. Focusing on your faults and shortcomings can lead to low self-esteem. You will undo this kind of thinking by concentrating more on the good points and characteristics.

CHAPTER FIVE

STEP BY STEP HYPNOTHERAPY FOR WEIGHT LOSS

With the fast rise in the number of people struggling to reach their targeted weight loss targets, another potential solution to overweight has emerged—efficient, result-oriented, and non-invasive weight loss hypnotherapy. One of the key reasons for its popularity is that the treatment does not require consulting consultants, purchasing vitamins, undertaking intense physical exercises, or even a low-carbon diet, etc. Hypnotherapy for weight loss may be conducted by a weight watcher-the most he or she may seek the aid of a skilled hypnotist. However, several may study and practice hypnotherapy at home via various self-help resources available.

Hypnotherapy for weight loss is not the only field in which hypnosis is used. It is pretty much recognized as one of the most viable treatment options for numerous mental and physical conditions, including pain control, depression, anxiety attacks, addictions, and many more. The effectiveness of the treatment option is demonstrated by the fact that even physicians now consider hypnotherapy to be a permanent loss of weight and refer their overweight patients to skilled hypnotists.

Losing weight by hypnosis can be achieved in two ways. The first approach is to see a licensed hypnotist who guides you through the process of hypnotism. However, the cost of care using the services of a hypnotist could be a deterrent to many. In such situations, you can take the second choice of self-hypnosis. There is no better help than self-help, after all.

Self-hypnosis is not a daunting activity, and there are numerous self-help methods, such as MP3 hypnosis, etc., that can be used to study and practice art in the comfort of your home. So, to shed those extra pounds, you don't have to go to the gym or buy those expensive diet pills. Hypnotherapy for weight loss has been shown to be successful, and there is no reason why it should not achieve the desired result for you.

The way hypnosis works are to lose weight by working at the subconscious level of the mind, the layer from which most of our cravings, phobias, fears, and apprehensions arise. Hypnosis is at the root of overeating, lack of motivation to perform physical activities, appetite for fried food, etc., by first soothing the mind and then injecting a variety of constructive ideas that the restful mind has taken up. Hypnotherapy for weight loss is so effective because it entirely changes the food thought. You become a more reasonable individual who can distinguish the good from the poor. You've turned into a more optimistic person who sets realistic weight loss goals and still succeeds.

Many people face weight loss issues that have not found a cure that will help them lose weight permanently. Supermarkets are now filled with protein drinks, diet pills, and other ridiculous food fads that have been launched by different business organizations just to get the attention of people who are overweight.

Out of desperation, these people often fall into the pit of patronizing any substance and not only lose weight but are victims of vicious side effects. This way is also to demonstrate that weight loss items are hyped up, and most of them have no significant or permanent impact. Thus, it is high time to find alternative weight loss methods and find Hypnotherapy for weight loss, which has been proven to be successful for millions of people around the world.

Practitioners have used hypnosis for many decades. As time passes, more and more research has shown that weight loss hypnotherapy is now accepted as one of the most successful methods of weight loss. Professional hypnotherapists can help people reach goals and objectives that previously seemed unlikely.

The rationale behind hypnosis is to infiltrate the patients' subconscious minds. No matter how much a person wishes to lose weight, but if they are not aware that their subconscious mind opposes him or her, it will never happen or will have considerable difficulty until the target is met. With the aid of a good hypnotist, constructive thoughts and ideas can be cultivated in the mind of the patient.

After hypnosis, when a patient resumes his or her regular life, their actions and habits are more concentrated on maintaining weight loss. This way dictates to the body what to do and how to react to such circumstances. If the patient dislikes exercise, it would not be an enjoyable and worthwhile thing for him or her to do even without supervision.

Fast and Naturally Loss of Weight with Hypnosis

Losing weight with hypnosis is one of the fastest, quickest, and safest and most calming and cheapest ways to lose weight permanently. I've been hypnotizing thousands of people for more than 17 years, and I haven't seen someone who tries to make this work fail for them when they try to do what they're supposed to do. There have been many independent studies on weight loss communities in many different ways, from medications to special diets, but none has performed as well as hypnosis. If you understand hypnosis and know what to expect, you're going to be effective in losing all the weight you want, and you need to lose, even if you don't believe it's going to work, it's going to work anyway. Hypnosis is working if you want it to work. Anyone can be hypnotized if they want to. You'll lose weight if you're going to lose weight. The only thing that can save you from being hypnotized is you. I've got people telling me, "I don't think I can be hypnotized." They're usually my best customers. They're usually people who have some significant myths about hypnosis and may have tried it, but nothing magical happened, so they gave up. They just want it to work, but they just didn't know how to do it until they were better informed about hypnosis.

There are some basic facts about hypnosis that you need to know is the right subject. When someone with experience hypnotizes you, you'll sit back and relax, close your eyes and listen to the hypnotherapist's voice to guide you. There's nothing you can do wrong; nothing can go wrong. There are no risks in this form of hypnosis. All hypnosis is self-hypnosis. You're still in charge of that. You're never going to do or say anything against your will, interests, values, or principles, regardless of what others think. It's like a mental test or a mind game. And you're not losing hold of your thoughts. You're still in charge of that. You're not losing your hearing or any of your senses. In reality, your senses become sharper, and you become more conscious, not less. You're still going to hear me whether you think you do it or not. You're doing all the work, and all the work is in your head. You don't have to say something or do something about it. The hypnotherapist uses their experience to guide you through your head, to send you guidance, but you don't have to follow them if you're not comfortable with any part of it. There's no sense of being hypnotized. You're not going to be hypnotized. The only thing you're going to experience is sort of comfortable to really comfortable. Others get just a little comfortable and listen to every word and remember it all, whereas others are so comfortable, they snorkel. Still, nobody can sleep until you're at home in bed for the night, and you're exhausted anyway when you put on your cd. Often it may feel like sleep, but it's not sleeping. All the work is in your head, so you have to take part and think about what the hypnotherapist suggests. It's just a guided meditation and incredibly strong.

With Hypnosis, you will be able to achieve your perfect weight and figure. You're going to lose all the weight you want and need to lose, without tension and emotional challenges with cravings, impulses, overfeeding, stuffing yourself as you do when you die. It's not a diet, but you're not going to put your weight back on! You don't feel like you're starving, though you're looking for more nutritious, lower-calorie, healthy foods. You won't want the rich, fattening, unhealthy, high calories, candy, unhealthy food, and food that isn't good for you. You're not going to snack or eat between meals or late at night. You're going to eat what your body wants, and when you're satisfied, you're fully satisfied. You won't lose weight as easily as it might damage your health. You will concentrate on the perfect shape and scale and achieve the ideal size quickly and without discomfort and keep that size as long as you want. You're going to want to drink more water and be happy from one meal to the next. You're going to lose weight without trying! Your eating habits can change suddenly, instantly, or gradually over time. Some people will be hypnotized once, and their eating habits will change forever, and others need to be hypnotized.

You use the subconscious mind, now more generally known as the higher self, higher consciousness, or super consciousness. It never rests more than the heart does. This way is where all of the control resides. You will learn to use the power inside guided meditation, and that is all it is guided meditation and very powerful meditation. It's best to get the hypnosis on a cd so that you can listen to it for 21 to 28 days as a booster. Some experts say that you need to listen to the hypnosis CD for 21 days to change your habits for a lifetime, while others say it takes 28 days. However, most people choose to listen to their CD for various reasons as there are so many benefits, whether for weight loss or otherwise. When you're hypnotized, it's a mental test, and you'll soon find that your memory improves. Your stress level is going down; you're going to sleep better and feel happy and healthier all the time. You can sense fresh and essential energy that flows through your body and mind every day that you wake up from a good night's rest with a more optimistic mindset. You will be more inspired than ever to workout, to take the time to be healthy every day. Ok, in my hypnosis anyway, you're going to gain from all this stuff when losing weight. Right hypnotherapy will always make you feel good, no matter what you're hypnotized for.

Rapid Weight Loss Risks

There are several risks associated with obesity. Heart disease, cholesterol, and diabetes are just some of the dangers of overweight. However, losing weight isn't the easiest thing to do. People with weight issues are continually losing their pounds and putting them on again. Is it any wonder that crash diets for rapid weight loss are becoming so popular? Rapid weight loss is something people's overweight are hoping for. But is there some fast weight loss program that could shave off the pounds and hold them off? What's more, losing weight is a super-fast idea? What are the health risks?

Yeah, these are some of the questions that should come to your mind when you look at commercials for fast weight loss programs. It could be tempting to look at a quick weight loss plan that means you're looking at a 20-pound slimmer reflection of yourself in a week, but don't give in to that temptation. The benefits of rapid weight loss may not be irreversible, and you may do irreparable harm to your metabolism. Thus, the positive effects can not last long, but the detrimental effects can end up haunting you forever.

If you are already susceptible to kidney issues, trying to lose weight quickly might make them worse. You can end up with gall bladder stones or low blood pressure, as well as mineral imbalances in your body. None of this will bode well for your wellbeing in the long run. Adding to this is the chance that you will regain all your lost weight within a few months of losing it. While some people profit from accelerated weight loss programs, the findings have not always favored the plan. Oprah Winfrey was a case in point a few years back when she woke us after losing weight to the oodles, but she put it all on again in a short time.

The quickest weight loss program appears to require you to starve yourself. This way is not the way to lose weight. Bear in mind that if you deprive yourself, you run the risk of binging yourself. So, you might end up eating a lot more than you've been dreaming about. The result: all the pounds you've lost will be back again. There is also a high risk that you will develop an eating disorder.

How do you plan to eradicate those pounds and hold them off? Eat right and exercise right. Many people prefer to go from overweight to slim to overweight again because they set unrealistic weight-loss expectations. The intention is to slow down but to keep going towards that objective. The quickest way to ensure that you do this is by adopting a healthy diet. Eat fats; eat carbohydrates; ingest those calories — just don't stuff yourself with them. Schedule yourself for a daily workout, drink a lot of water, and have a nice rest. Soon, you should be looking at a slimmer you minus the consequences of a rapid weight loss.

Being overweight is something that almost any person in the world is trying to stop. This way is incredibly right given the number of health hazards that one is exposed to while he or she is overweight and the issues with self-esteem that come with not being in shape. It is, therefore, not shocking that weight-loss diets and fat loss exercises are standard in the world today. However, to shed extra fat, some people typically use techniques that help them lose weight fast, which is generally to the detriment of their bodies. The following are the hazards to which one is subjected as he or she attempts to lose weight quickly.

It is usually recommended that one should make sure that he or she does not lose more than 2 lbs a week. Any weight loss of more than 2 lbs. is generally considered risky as it typically exposes a person's body to significant health risks. This way is because rapid fat loss typically denies the body the time it requires to adapt to weight loss and therefore creates instability in the body's metabolic system, which can often have disastrous implications.

Rapid weight loss can lead to muscle and organ tissue breakdown, which can adversely affect your overall health. Some fat loss diets designed to induce rapid weight loss typically lead to extreme protein deficiency in the body of a person. Since amino acids are critical when it comes to muscle regeneration and boosting the immune system, the body may be forced to use proteins that shape organs and other muscle tissues, causing a lot of health problems.

The use of diets designed to induce rapid weight loss is likely to put you at risk of osteoporosis. This fact is incredibly right if the main diet is deficient in calcium when you lose weight. As a result, the bones can grow fragile and become vulnerable to fractures. It is also essential to be cautious when you start to lose weight more quickly, as this can also suggest that your bones are getting weaker in the process.

Rapid weight loss, too, puts the heart at risk of failure. This way is because rapid weight shifts typically do not allow the heart enough time to adapt to changing circumstances. As a consequence, rapidly gaining weight or naturally losing weight creates increased stress on the heart muscles. Increased pressure can also lead to heart failure.

The wonder of Slimming Hypnosis

What would you think if you could use the power of your own mind to create weight loss? No more weight loss books, no more diets. And more importantly, there's no sense of remorse if you indulge in the forbidden!

It's conceivable. You can as well make use of the power of your mind to think yourself thin. By seeing yourself slimmer and thought thinner, you are conditioning the subconscious mind to bring about a change in eating habits. This way is it-no trickery, no magic pills. Hypnosis is being used to demonstrate how the ability to see yourself as you want to be can be programmed and thus achieved. All you have to do is to believe in yourself simply, and that change is possible.

What's the term that comes to mind when you try to squeeze into a dress for a date, and you are unable to pull up the zipper or the buttons are so stretched, they could pop. You know you think, "I'm so fat; I don't want to be fat anymore"-the word fat needs to be eliminated from your vocabulary. Why? Because when you use the word fat, your subconscious mind thinks "okay, fat = cream cakes, chocolate, etc." so you have set up a negative thought process. On the other hand, "I want to be slimmer" is more positive because the subconscious mind now has to think "what is slim, slimmer = better food choices, exercise."

How many times did you eat something fattening and ask, "Why did I eat that?" With hypnosis, you become more conscious of what you're eating. A motto like "I can take it, or I can leave it because I'd rather leave it" to give you power. You've made a choice that you just don't want to eat. It's all about getting to listen to your body. What does your body want? When pregnant, people give in to their cravings because they feel that the baby needs it. Watch kids; they eat what they want when they want it.

The purpose of using hypnosis is to break the emotional bond with food. Part of this method is to imagine yourself as you want to see be-to yourself slim. Thinking thin contributes to the concept of thinking like a thin person. I can take it or leave it, and I'd instead leave it. Do I really want this right now? Is it my mood? What caused my mood? So, looking at the emotion that influences the reaction to eat.

The following little exercise is a perfect way to teach yourself the strength of your mind and how it can affect your decisions.

Take a deep breath, hold on to the mental count of 4, and let go of the breath. Do these two more times and softly close your eyes on the 3rd round.

Count it down from 1 to 10.

Tense and loosen the muscles from the toes and legs and work to the very top of your head.

Think of the words "calm and comfortable."

Imagine a table full of all the food and drink you know is bad for you. Notice the fullness of the food and the different shades of brown.

There is an incinerator near the table, and it is on fire and ready for use.

Now you've thrown all the food and drink from the table into the incinerator-all the food and drink you know is bad for you.

When the table is clear, see all the food you can eat and know the water-notice all the bright colors, and feel the warmth coming from the food.

Now, put a frame around the photo and place a big tick next to it. This sign is a demonstration to your subconscious mind that these are the foods you now like.

Now see yourself as you want to be, smaller, more formal, more fabulous.

Place this picture next to the good food.

Keep this picture, and where do you feel good about this picture. Note in your body, is it your head, your chest, your stomach, and make you feel bigger, lighter, and full of color.

Feel great

Count from 10 to 1 and return to full consciousness. Take a moment to entirely focus yourself and take stock of the picture of healthy, vibrant food and water and the beautiful image of yourself as you should be as you become.

So, think yourself thin and see yourself thin, look at the hypnosis to grow this picture.

CHAPTER SIX

THE EFFECTIVE METHOD OF LOSING WEIGHT HEALTHILY IN LESS THAN 10 DAYS

People on the heavier side of the scale frequently see weight loss targets as a nightmare. Well, guy! The good news is, it's not as hard as you think it's going to be. All it takes is commitment and dedication to carry out your weight loss plans. Strong exercise and malnutrition are not the best way to think about your waistline. You have to be careful about what you feed your body in terms of food, exercise, and behaviors.

Here are a few tips that will help you begin to lose weight in just 10 days.

1. Drink more of the water

Drink enough water, up to 8 glasses a day, to keep the body hydrated. Water has an important role to play in the weight loss plan. It's the easiest detoxifying agent that flushes toxins out of your body. Drinking water before meals often allows you to feel full sooner.

2. Smaller servings of food

Prepare a list of the necessary nutrients that you need to provide to your body. Now split them into smaller portions of meals to be eaten during the day. This way, you're not going to under nourish yourself and allow your system time to digest food on time.

3. Please say no to fast food

Sacrificing your favorite food for quite a while could tempt you to eat junk food. One simpler way to do this is to keep your kitchen free from clutter to make it unavailable. Another approach is to educate yourself about the adverse effects that it has on your health. These foods are made of empty calories with little nutritional value whatsoever.

4. Cut the Calories down

The golden rule for weight loss is to eat more calories than you consume. Check the calorie content of a food item and its nutritional value. Unused calories are going to be stored as fat in your body.

5. Limit the intake of sugar, carbs, and sodium

Not all carbohydrates are unhealthful, make sure you stick to only safe and more natural carbohydrates. Sugar is a delicious poison high in calories for those with weight loss plans. Salt has a water retention attribute that just adds to your weight.

6. Eat Lean Protein

The proteins are the main building blocks of the muscles. It retains muscle strength even though you lose weight. They also help you lose weight faster as muscles require constant energy, which keeps fat burning even during sleep. Stick to make lean protein options like fish, chicken, beans, and lentils.

7. Depend on Whole Grains and Fiber

Whole grains and fiber-rich food can help you remain full for longer. This way avoids mid-meal snacks and weight loss aids. It also increases healthy cholesterol and regulates poor levels of cholesterol. Furthermore, these foods have very low-calorie content.

8. Replace all food packets with new food

Packed foods contain high levels of sugar, carbs, and fat. Instead of storing your shelf with packaged food products, go for greens and sprouts. They are healthier in-between meals with a much higher nutritional value.

9. To stay physically involved

Forming habits that stimulate physical activity is a positive indicator. Instead, use your tea break for a fast stroll. Miss the elevators and use the stairs. Enable yourself to do things that improve your cardio. All of these improvements will lead to more calories being consumed than before.

10. Eat it slowly

Chew the food. Not only does this ease digestion, but it also sends a signal of satiety to the brain. This way is going to keep a check on feeding.

11. Drink a green teacup

Drinking green tea instead of traditional tea and coffee is a perfect way to help with weight loss. It detoxifies the body and is lower in calories than regular tea.

12. Making a walk in your habit

Give yourself a chance to walk the extra mile whenever possible. Maybe indoor or outdoor, walking is going to have its health benefits. It re-energizes your aerobic exercise and helps you consume more calories.

13. Evite Alcohol

If you want to lose weight, stay away from alcohol. Alcohol follows unsanitary snacking and gives the body no nutritional benefit.

14. Drink soft honey lime and cinnamon water

You may not like it as much as your favorite carbonated soda. Yet it has tremendous health benefits. Drinking this in the morning daily for 10 days is sure to lose a few extra pounds. It also removes the body from toxins. Plus, it doesn't sell any empty calories like your artificial sweetened drinks.

15. Shape a routine of exercise

Good eating is just as important, so it is a daily exercise. It stimulates your metabolism and keeps you healthy. Full body exercise is very useful for overall health, but you can start with simple cardio, skipping, or jogging. It uses up the calories it absorbs.

16. Never combine food with other things

If you're eating while watching TV or gossip with your friends, you're likely to eat unintentionally. This way adds unnecessary calories that you could have stopped.

17. Socialize with people who are physically fit

Keep your social circle in bloom with fitness freaks. This way will keep your spirits up and encourage you to share useful fitness ideas.

18. Read the food labels

Ok, know your supermarket. Read the labels of the product to find the nutritional value that it provides. Understanding what is right and wrong for your wellbeing will help you pick your grocery store wisely.

19. Have a sound of sleep

Sleep well for at least 7 to 8 hours, so you're able to face the challenges of the next day. Sleeping also regulates and activates the appetite hormones ghrelin and leptin. Also, if you're up until late in the night, you'll end up eating unhealthful and readily available snacks.

20. Keep motivated and stick to your goals

One significant weakness in people's weight loss strategies is that they do not abide by the rules and targets. To reap its rewards, you must be determined towards your goals. Over time, don't let your inspiration slip away.

When you're trying to lose weight, it's tempting to want results as fast as possible.

Yet quickly losing weight is unlikely to help you keep your weight off – and it also comes with health risks. If you are putting efforts and trying to lose weight, you would want to see and feel a difference quickly. It may be tempting to trust one of the many plans that promise a fast, easy weight loss.

Unfortunately, even if these diets help you lose weight, you cannot maintain a healthy weight for months and years to come. The most effective method to lose weight and hold it off is to lose weight steadily. This method may involve implementing a weight loss plan, but it should also include making adjustments to your diet and activity levels that you can commit to for the long term. Weight loss appears to level off for a while, and you may need to make more adjustments. If you're struggling to get a healthy weight after attempting a healthy eating plan, talk to your GP or nurse for advice. You can also consult with your GP if you have a long-term health problem before starting a diet.

Secure rates of weight loss

If you're trying to lose weight, the healthy weekly weight loss range is between 0.5 kg and 1 kg. It's between 1 lb. and 2 lb. a week. Lose weight quicker than this, and you are at risk for health issues that include malnutrition and gallstones and feeling exhausted and unwell. Fad diets associated with speedy weight loss, which entail merely changing the diet for a few weeks, are often unlikely to lead to a healthier weight in the long run.

Find out how much weight you really need to lose and get a personal daily calorie range to keep up with our healthy weight calculator. Beware of purchasing counterfeit or unlicensed medicinal items marketed as slimming goods. Get in touch and see what you're getting.

Eat Healthy and Sleep Better with Hypnosis

Hypnosis can conjure up visions of people being made to quack like a duck on stage, but the fact is that it's usually much more boring — and sleep-inducing. Correct, hypnosis can be a valuable technique for certain people dealing with some sleeping conditions, such as insomnia or sleepwalking.

For people with insomnia, hypnosis can help both the body and the mind relax and let go of the anxiety that cannot be triggered by falling asleep. A sleepwalker, on the other hand, can learn to wake up when his feet touch the floor with a hypnotic suggestion. Hypnosis can also increase the amount of time you spend in slow sleep (deep sleep) by as much as 80%. This fact is crucial because deep sleep is vital for memory and healing so that you can wake up feeling refreshed.

Unlike what you would expect, hypnosis doesn't happen when you watch a swinging pocket watch. It's typically achieved by listening to the verbal signals of a hypnotherapist who pulls you into a trance-like state that could be likened to being so engrossed in a good book that you're blocking out your surroundings. For example, a session aimed at helping you sleep more deeply is likely to involve a soft, calming voice using words like "relax," "deep," "easily," and "let go." Afterward, or even while listening, you could drift to sleep. Although some people interpret being hypnotized as feeling incredibly calm, the brain is intensely concentrated during hypnotism.

Hypnotherapy may work better for some people. That's because certain people are more "suggested" than others — that is, they're more easily drawn into a hypnotized state. Around a fifth of people, however, actually cannot be hypnotized.

Are you interested in trying it? People who use hypnosis to help overcome usually sleep issues see results after only a few sessions, so you don't have to make a significant commitment. Hypnotherapy is not a stand-alone cure for sleep problems, but rather a method to try, which is also performed by physicians, nurses, which psychotherapists. Talk to your doctor for a referral.

You should skip grains and stop drinking, and put chia seeds in your oats and exercise, and do all the hard, dull, will-powerful things that people do to lose weight. You should fight your impulses, get rid of your habits, and slowly, painfully grind your excess fat out of life.

Or maybe you should just ... You want less food. This way is the fundamental concept behind weight-loss hypnotherapy: it couldn't be simpler. You just go to a couple of meetings, and then you don't have to combat temptation at all, because you don't even notice it. It sounds pretty nice for a life untroubled by the allure of sugar.

By inducing a state of suggestive relaxation-hypnosis-in the patient, say the practitioners, which helps them to reprogram the unconscious mind. The patient, contrary to common opinion, will remain awake and alert, recalling the session. The doctor would not use a softly swinging pocket watch. Patients must want care to succeed.

What is it used for?

In addition to weight loss, hypnotherapy is also used to treat addictions, improve habits, alleviate anxiety, and relieve pain.

And is it working?

As the skeptics' encyclopedia Logical Wiki put it, "is not generally accepted as a primary treatment by the medical and psychological community." It's easy to find anecdotal proof for it, but it's just as easy to see examples of its failure. Various studies show the efficacy of hypnotherapy in the treatment of a variety of conditions, especially pain. However, it is far from uniformly accurate and relies heavily on the patient's ability to do so. It can never be used as a replacement for evidence-based medicines.

Doctors are struggling for weight control in the front lines. They have the thankless duty of convincing their patients that they are overweight and, in many cases, obese. Impressing them that they can only feel better and live longer is to keep the weight under control. We all know these things; we just find it too difficult to change our habits.

You may already have specific health concerns associated with becoming overweight, such as high cholesterol and high triglycerides. You may have symptoms of diabetes, cardiac, or thyroid conditions, not to mention digestive and respiratory issues. These things aren't going to grow overnight. They are long-term diseases and disorders that can be avoided.

Why do we want to do the same thing when faced with our health and the bad choices we've made? People talk about making the required improvements, and I can only speak for myself when I say that I just want to do better at the time. So why are we going to fail, again and again? It's time to come up with some answers and change the course of your life.

The answers are in your mind, as I said before. Deep in the unconscious mind, you will find the source of low self-esteem and self-confidence. Messages you've heard and internalized over and over since childhood, without even understanding it. All nutritional attempts and weight loss fail miserably, and more weight is always added.

The most powerful way to get through your conscious mind and into your subconscious mind is by subliminal programming. Completely healthy and free from physical side effects, all you need to do is relax and listen to the embedded optimistic messages that are played along with soft music. It's like you're floating on a moon!

Your conscious mind, which would usually jump in to fight positive signals with negative thoughts, is profoundly relaxed during the process. This fact allows signs to go straight to the subconscious part of the brain where they are recognized as real.

Our lives are full of subliminal messages. Much of this is something we cannot manage, and yet these messages have the ability to have a drastic effect on our lives, that they're doing! You will feel much happier when you begin to fill your subconscious mind with safe, optimistic, constructive messages.

Your life will get better and better as you step forward and make the improvements you need and eventually drop those extra pounds. The secret to weight loss success is re-programming your mind with hypnosis and subliminal programming.

Learn to Eat Mindfully through Meditation and Simple Habits

For most people, the dream of losing weight seems to entail a lifetime of misery and hardship, most often with nothing to show for it other than an intense feeling of disappointment. That's going to end for you now. Here you can learn how to combine the power of mindfulness of your diet with the use of hypnosis. This manner is to put the exhausting cycle to an end once and for all so that you lose weight and become the slim that you have been looking for. As someone once opined, "Nothing tastes as Good as Slimness," and that's so real, don't you think?

Creating a Healthy Body Takes Commitment

Most certainly, you already know what food is right for you, what food is not, and what bad eating habits you have that lead to your weight gain and your weight loss becoming more balanced and happier. Yet, you will feel like you lack the "willpower" to lose weight and hold it off. It's not the will power you need. You just need a bit of help in bringing your subconscious mind on board to make a meaningful change, and you need to learn a few basic tactics that will help you on the path to success. Through reading this chapter, you have shown that you are willing to commit to look and sound at your best. No matter how much you've weighed or where you live, you can be saved.

Mindfully Eating Leads to Success

Overweight? Overweight? You're overeating and you're filling! It means you're eating way more than your body needs to keep it going. Assuming that your doctor has found you safe, with no metabolic problems, the simple truth is that you need to eat less garbage and more protein to lose and then sustain your weight.

The major problem with many people in today's fast-paced, fast-food world is that we're eating away too much, not consciously mindful of what we're doing. Studies have shown that this kind of eating allows us to consume much more than we would usually do, so we neglect or refuse to understand the signals of our bodies that we are full. As a result, the first step in your determination to lose weight needs to become more conscious of your diet.

Mindfulness (which has its origins in Buddhism) is a term that psychologists have invented to mean that you are deliberately paying attention to your behavior. Many people seem to go through a lot of life being unmindful, not paying attention to the world around them, or consuming. So, being aware of your behavior is key to curbing your eating and making you safe. Eating is mindful of the use of mindfulness meditation. Mindfulness focuses our attention and knowledge on the "now" that, in turn, helps us detach from our usual, unproductive behaviors and activities. Mindful eating at every meal allows one to explore a more satisfying connection to eating and nutrition than we have ever known. There is a kind of nourishment that provides fulfillment at a profound emotional level. Note that obesity also has an emotional aspect to it. And how are we going to do this mindful eating?

Being diligent and intentionally eating is as easy as it sounds; you need to be mindful of your eating. This fact means that when you're feeding, that's What you're doing: providing. You're not watching TV, reading a newspaper, or checking your Facebook profile. You eat, paying attention to the scent, colors, taste, and texture of each bite. Enjoy the meal. There are a few things that happen when you're aware of your eating habits: you enjoy your meal more, you feel satisfied more easily, and you make healthier choices on what to eat. Here's a short guide on how to eat:

Build a calm and enjoyable atmosphere in which to feed. Don't eat in front of the TV or at your desk at work. So you end up screwing your food down with no respect or knowledge of what you're consuming. Before you hit the biscuit, ask yourself: how do you feel? Are you relaxed, nervous, bored, or maybe even feeling depressed? (Are you thirsty rather than hungry? Often the two feelings are confused). Just understand and acknowledge the sensation, whatever it might be, and then analyze your stomach: how does it feel? It's easier to digest food and be careful when you're comfortable. When we recognize our feelings, they seem to leave us feeling calmer and less likely to pick up a biscuit (or only one won't hurt).

Chew your meal, slow down! It takes at least 20 minutes for your brain to register your stomach full. If you continue eating till you feel full, you're basically "overfull" or more colloquially "stuffed," and that's not mindful of eating. Take your time, enjoy and savor every bite. Note the temperature, scent, texture, and taste of each morsel of food you put (not shovel) in your mouth. Note how much more relaxed the stomach feels when the food is chewed thoroughly. This fact also makes it easier for the digestive system too. Note how much more fulfilled you are when you take the time to enjoy and savor every bite of your meal. I sometimes refer to a fuel gauge as a reference to when to feed and when to avoid eating.

Never allow yourself to get empty below "3" and stop eating when you get full to "7." If you eat until the gauge reads "10" you're going to overeat. When serving your meal, choose a smaller plate and, as a result, reduce the size of your serving. But don't despair, because now that you're eating thoughtfully, you're going to feel as full and as odd as it may sound as if you were using a larger plate. Try to leave a little portion of food on your plate when you hit 7 out of 10. You will have to silence the "mother voice" in your head about "eating everything on your plate."

It is also critical that you have a decent amount of protein in your food choices, and that you 'graze' about six meals a day with a 'snack' protein every second meal. So, there's an overview here. You can master the mindfulness of eating in two ways. Next, keep a diary of food. A food diary will help you recognize trends in your eating and recognize when you may eat out of anger rather than starvation. It will even help you see if you're overeating junk food and a lack of healthy food.

Be mindful of what you're doing when, when, and how you're eating what you're eating. Mindful eating is the first step in the path to weight loss and maintenance. The next move is as follows:

Hypnosis: Makes Healthy Mindful Eating Easy

You've committed yourself when you're ready to eat thoughtfully and genuinely alleviate your excess weight. You will worry that you won't be able to conquer your cravings and the various temptations of modern, culinary life on your own, and you're probably correct. But don't worry-hypnosis can help.

A qualified, professional hypnotist will work with you to stop your cravings and ensure your continued weight loss success. Although hypnosis is not magic, some people believe it operates mystically, and they are surprised at the results they achieve effortlessly. While you're in hypnosis, the hypnotist can speak directly to your subconscious, remember the difficulties you've had with losing weight in the past, and the unhealthy patterns that have formed after. The hypnotist would tell your subconscious to liberate you from cravings, fear, and harmful decisions, and inspire your subconscious to make good dietary choices. When you recover from hypnosis, you may not feel anything other than a little relaxed. Yet you will instantly note the difference in your cravings. You would no longer want salt, candy, or any of your other indulgences. Instead, the body needs to eat nutritious foods in the right proportions. With the power of hypnosis working and your determination and awareness of the need to eat wisely, you can find the path to your ideal weight and the simple way to walk. Start relieving weight today. No matter where you're living, You can do it most effectively with the aid of someone trained in the art of hypnosis.

Overcoming Binge Eating

Overcoming binge eating with hypnosis is a simple, natural approach that can help you fight munchies. Instead of attempting to push yourself to abstain from what you feel compelled to do, through hypnosis, you may use the aid of your subconscious mind.

First of all and foremost, we must have a good understanding of what we're talking about. So, what exactly does the binge eat? It's an eating disorder that often causes a person to consume a lot of food in a short time. It doesn't matter whether or not the person is hungry-they just keep eating and eating.

Hypnosis is essentially a mental procedure that puts you in a very calm state of mind that makes it easier to make a personal improvement decision. If you use hypnosis to resolve binge eating, you can either visit a hypnotherapist or use a pre-recorded hypnotic induction specially made for binge eating. There is no way to tell which is the best choice-what matters is that you have an excellent hypnotist and that the pre-recorded hypnotic induction is produced by an accomplished professional.

It typically takes two to eight weeks of daily hypnotic relaxation for this to take effect. There are many things you can do to make binge eating treatment even more successful. Take a notebook and a pen, for example, and start writing a "binge journal." In this diary, you write when you figured out, what happened before, and what kind of thoughts and feelings you had before the show.

This writing of a binge journal will help you better understand the psychological patterns that underlie your eating disorder and determine what causes it. Then you should think of ways to stop the causes.

Often, make sure you're consuming many small meals all day, and don't want to starve yourself. The hungrier you are, the more likely you will be to indulge yourself in binge eating again.

If necessary, include a friend, a family member, or a coach. This fact should be a person you can either call or even visit when you feel like another episode is coming. Just speak to this person about your feelings and emotions, which will help you fight the urge a little better.

You don't have to do all of these things. Overcoming binge eating with hypnosis works very effectively-but; the more actively you get involved in the process, the quicker you get through it.

A lot of people are overweight just because they are emotionally reliant on food. If you're one of them, you know what it feels like. This box of cookies is not just a delicious treat; instead, it is a strong addiction that fills an emotional gap.

How do you know if you're addicted to food?

Tell yourself the following questions:

- Do you think you're worried about food?

- Are you going to eat binges that you can't control and that you feel bad about later?

- Do you want to eat when things get complicated, like when you're stressed out or depressed?

If you replied "yes" to all of these questions, the relationship between your emotions and food is not a good one.

So, what if you're addicted to food? Are you out of luck?

No, not!

You can get rid of your emotional dependency on food by losing weight with hypnosis.

You've got to be careful how you're going to handle a food problem. After all, you can't stop eating "cold turkey" like you can try to do with cigarettes or alcohol. You need food to survive, but you also need healthier eating habits so that you can regulate your consumption of food-not the other way around.

The disappointing news is that you can't do it all by yourself. The good news is that a hypnotist and weight loss hypnosis experts will improve.

It's not what you think when you take a picture of a magician standing on the stage, waving a watch and making people cluck like chickens. Instead, actual weight loss hypnosis has a lot of evidence to back it up!

Your emotional dependency on food is in the depths of your subconscious mind. Somehow, your subconscious has come up with the notion that food is the only way to make you feel better. Instead of dwelling on the destructive emotions surrounding you, you're concentrating your attention on how good food tastes. You don't have to experience something terrible like that.

If you lose weight with hypnosis, you will be in a trance-like state, where you will be open to suggestions. From there, you can train your subconscious mind to concentrate on other tasks when things get difficult instead of eating. You might train your subconscious to take a walk around the block when you get stressed out or to close your eyes and take a few deep breaths when you get sad.

By educating your subconscious in this way, you're giving it a better option for coping. Soon enough, you will know that you want food for what it is-a a delicious treat-instead of an emotional crutch!

CHAPTER SEVEN

POSITIVE STATEMENTS FOR WEIGHT LOSS

We seem to underestimate how strong our minds are and fail to make full use of their ability. Your subconscious mind will believe everything you think, and it can be trained to succeed.

If your subconscious mind joins, it can affect your actions and what you can do. One way you can prepare your mind for weight loss success is by positive affirmations.

What Are Positive Affirmations?

Positive claims are strong words that we reinforce to ourselves (either in our mind or out loud) and are usually things we want to do. They are used to develop our inner thought and affect our actions and the performance we experience. Say them regularly with confidence and true conviction, and then your subconscious mind will come to embrace them as truth. This way will strengthen your new optimistic self-image and charge you with positive energy. When your mind begins to accept that something is real, your mindset, actions, and thought can change and bring about a positive change. Positive affirmations may be tailored to any aim you wish to accomplish, including weight loss.

Reasonable assertions for weight loss

You need to use a handful of optimistic claims about weight loss that will inspire you and show what you want to achieve.

Here are some suggestions for constructive assertions about weight loss: -

- Losing weight comes easily to me.

- I'm going to meet my weight loss goals.

- I lose weight every day.

- I love the taste of nutritious foods.

- I'm in control of how much I eat.

- I love to practice; it makes me feel perfect.

- I'm getting fitter and stronger through exercise.

- I build more balanced eating habits all the time.

- I'm getting slimmer every day.

- I look fine, and I feel amazing.

Try and use positive statements that make you feel comfortable working for you. You have to tell them regularly (at least 3-4 times a day) with a real conviction for them to do. Often tell them when you wake up in the morning and the last thing before bed. If you can find time alone, it can be very inspiring to say it out loud. Write down your optimistic affirmations on a card and bring them around with you at any time of the day for an immediate boost. You might also post it to your refrigerator, a perfect way to make you think about it before you snack.

You have to say you're positive statements regularly (each day) for at least 30 days to build a habit. It's also essential that you get into the habit of ejecting unpleasant habits when they invade your brain. Use positive affirmations for weight loss success every day, look forward to a new look, and keep you well.

If you are worried about your weight, whether for cosmetic or medical purposes, and are motivated to get back in shape, there are various ways to do this. Many people try strict eating plans and exercise programs, but if this sounds all too familiar, you may find it helpful to learn how to use hypnosis for weight loss.

Hypnotherapy can be a powerful tool; it can almost immediately encourage you to change your attitude about food and eating forever. Hypnosis happens when the state of consciousness changes; many professionals are now providing programs in this area that help people break habits and addictions.

Proponents of these strategies say that they can be used to alleviate cravings and become more self-confident. While the medical community may indicate that hypnotherapy alone does not cure obesity, the findings may suggest that the reverse is valid.

Until you decide to work with a hypnotist to try to form yourself, you should make an effort to find a professional who is experienced in this sector. A typical hypnotist does not have the expertise and skills to make a difference, which is why it is essential to take the time to find a person who has the requisite know-how and, if possible, how skilled in weight loss.

You may as well be wondering how a hypnotist can bring about such a positive change. When you are under hypnosis, the psychiatrist will put ideas and thoughts in your subconscious mind that affect the way you think about food while you are awake. For example, phrases such as "snacking are not appealing to you; consuming vegetables is more desirable to you than junk food." These statements are going to get stuck in your head and enable you to maintain healthy eating habits.

It is normal to be a little apprehensive while deciding whether to use hypnotherapy to achieve your goals. It is imperative to clearly state that this is a healthy practice and is now embraced in mainstream society. The decision to use hypnosis should be made with a strong and relaxed mind, and after having already pursued other weight-loss plans.

It takes practice to trigger an immediate change in your mind from negative to positive. Be a Master to eliminate negative thoughts, opinions, discussions, and acts as soon as possible would dramatically increase your weight loss success or any other success in your life.

Why the tools?

- Reduce the "noise" in your head
- Decrease / remove negative trends of experience
- Disrupt the normal negative habit
- Decrease / Remove Apprehension
- Shift / Expand your perception;
- Increase / accelerate results
- Detox the feelings

Gratitude Tool-If you're centered and often obsessed with losing weight, you may forget to be grateful for who you are right now.

There are many ways to practice appreciation every day in your life. One approach is to write 1 to 3 items that you are thankful for at the end of the day in a personal Appreciation Journal. It's a perfect opportunity to do this right before you fall asleep. Gratitude is the last thing your brain recalls until you slip into a deep, restful sleep.

Receive Tool-It's essential to be able to obtain your new beautiful ideal body in several ways. If you don't get it in the smallest of ways, you won't receive it in significant ways.

The most critical incentive for weight loss performance is: completely accept who you are right now. Remember when you are not, and use the Reset Method to re-program your mind.

Reset Tool-Use this tool right after you encounter negative feelings, opinions, interactions, or behavior. Seconds after the unpleasant moment, say "reset" aloud (or in silence, considering the situation). Replace the negative with a potent argument. A general statement that you can speak to reset at any moment would be, "I chose strong thoughts and beliefs!"

Daily Meditation for Weight Loss

People are still looking for a reason to lose weight. They always enjoy finding ways to lose weight in the fastest way in the shortest time possible, yet they always end up in disappointment. Nowadays, yoga seems to be the most common type of weight loss exercise since people say it's very easy to practice, and there's no noise when you start doing yoga. Yoga asanas will be one of the most common forms of yoga. Yoga asanas for weight loss are becoming a favorite subject among yoga practitioners. It will be a matter of time before yoga asanas for weight loss are practiced across the world!

How does it work? When practicing asana yoga, concentrate on how you feel physically. As a first rule, don't care about feeling the pain to see the impact. Remember the saying, "No pain, no benefit" This is the moment you're going to get to see it! Whenever you start to lose weight with yoga asanas, you will begin to see positive changes within your body as you start to lose all the excess weight from your body. Feel every movement of your body whenever you can as you do yoga, as this puts you in sync with your body. When you're doing yoga, it's also a good idea to listen to calming and soothing music to help you concentrate when you're doing your daily yoga meditation. Listen to your body, too; you can stop and rest when you're tired. A tired body isn't good at doing yoga, and you're going to do yourself a favor if you relax first before resuming yoga asanas for weight loss.

Weight Loss: The Ayurvedic Route

For millions of Americans, Ayurvedic weight loss solutions have components for burning the excess fat that diet plans fail to answer. The problem with many food strategies and fads is that they do not consider the essential characteristics of the human body. The three elements, or dosha, of the body emphasized by Ayurvedic medicine must be placed in complete harmony to get rid of excess fat and generally remain healthy. The Kasha Dosha constitution focuses on the components of the body of the earth. Casha imbalance also contributes to obesity, high blood pressure, hypertension, heart disease, and the risk of organ failure.

Many on the Ayurvedic diet lose weight not through counting calories or missing food, but by relying on the ability of Ayurvedic weight loss recipes to reconfigure damaged body elements. Though kasha dosha is most likely a cause of weight concern, it is not rare for other body types to encounter difficulties in maintaining a healthy body structure.

The pitta aspect is that of fire, which is used to burn energy derived from your diet. Naturally, failure to properly process food in the pitta dosha would result in too much energy stored in the form of fat on your body. Likewise, vata dosha usually results in trim and balanced body figures. Still, consuming too much risky food for this body type will reverse the normal metabolism and build up body fat clumps.

The Ayurvedic way of losing weight focuses on many different aspects of everyday life. Ayurvedic medicine maintains that several additional steps can be taken on the road to healthy living instead of merely trimming down on portion size, eliminating carbohydrates, or intensifying exercises. This way involves a regular diet and exercise and meditation, massage, oil therapy, grooming, and spiritual fulfillment. After all, there is no point in reducing the calories of your daily meals if you lack self-discipline and determination to see it through and maintain a balanced lifestyle.

People utilizing these Ayurvedic diet methods lose weight by various means, but the Ayurvedic herbal approach is often the most effective. Certain herbs increase the pitta factor within — even for body types that are not usually strongly associated with pitta dosha — which results in greater metabolic ability, more energy during the day, improved blood circulation, and eventually more fat being processed by the body. Ginger may be the essential herb; those following Ayurvedic treatments lose weight at a much faster rate when they drink two to three cups of ginger tea a day in addition to a small amount of ginger before meals. Not only does the herb cause pitta to burn at a higher rate, but it temporarily limits the taste buds, suppresses the appetite, and allows less food to be consumed.

Spicy herbs such as cumin, black pepper, cinnamon, mustard seed, and cayenne are all highly recommended in Ayurvedic weight loss recipes. Like ginger, a spicy herb can serve as an acceleration of the metabolic process. These spices contain a form of oil that causes the body to have a higher function when released. Digestion acts faster to process fat, as the heart pumps more blood to stimulate the sweat glands and release heat. As such, spicy food acts as a miniature exercise, causing a part of the meal to be burned in consuming it!

The ease of losing weight by fad diets is not working for a long time. Almost 100 percent of dietary plans have failed over a decade. However, adopting an Ayurvedic diet can turn not only your body but also your energy levels and your everyday life. Ayurvedic weight loss remedies concentrate on the food process through pitta dosha. Addressing imbalances or accelerating a dosha will keep the body's natural elements balanced and in harmony.

Weight loss appears to be a matter of concern to many people at some stage in their lives. The first line of action to get rid of the dreaded extra pounds is diet and exercise. Currently, there may be hundreds of services aimed at helping you lose weight, but keeping ahead of both weight loss plans and fitness initiatives is always a difficult challenge.

The values and feelings that we subconsciously carry about ourselves decide our reality and the outcome that we encounter in our lives. We describe ourselves using our values and their complement. To bring about improvements in our experience, we need to decide which subconscious values need to shift and make specific beneficial changes. Hypnosis and meditation are a perfect technique for this purpose.

Now, you can keep up with your goals and commit to maintaining a positive lifestyle by incorporating hypnosis with your diet and exercise routine to meet your weight loss goals. A healthy diet is a key to weight loss, but life always gets in the way, the tension and tension of your history and everyday activities can easily lead you back to unhealthful eating habits. But hypnosis will help you handle this by pushing you to reach into your subconscious to tackle the feelings that make you continue to indulge. Better eating habits will then emerge from your new understanding of yourself and the reasons for your bad food choices. As a result, the nutritional component of your weight loss strategy will become tangible.

Exercise is often seen as the most unattainable target of any weight loss strategy. Still, it is incredibly important to start exercising as soon as a balanced diet becomes the norm. The benefits of physical exercise are frequently extolled, but as helpful as you know it to be, working out in a gym by yourself can be overwhelming because it often seems like someone else is making more progress than you do. Hypnosis, too, may help shed light on your problems, such as feeling insecure or low self-esteem, in order to build trust and encourage you to optimize the impact of your healthy diet and contribute to positive weight-loss trends and happier life.

Hypnosis is then the secret to opening the door to a dramatically improved lifestyle. You may say "good riddance" to crash diets, event diets, and other short programs with intense improvements in eating and practicing habits to attend an event hoping for the acceptance of others. Hypnosis can allow you to believe that real progress is the product of introspection.

So, the next move is to select a diet and exercise routine that works for you. It is often recommended that you visit a doctor who can also suggest potential weight-loss diets and physical fitness programs that will place you on the right road to improvement that will last for the rest of your life.

What's Meditation?

Meditation is a regular activity that involves clearing your mind so that you can return to a position of thought and relaxed emotions. Some people exercise for just five minutes a day, but most meditation experts recommend practicing for up to 20 minutes a day.

Meditation doesn't have to be challenging to do. If you're just starting, try to take five minutes as soon as you wake up to clear your mind before you face a busy day. Just close your eyes and focus on the rhythm of your breathing without attempting to alter it. Just concentrate on your breathing. If your mind wanders — and possibly at first — just direct it back to your breathing without judgment.

While Libshtein recommends training for 10 minutes a day (five minutes in the morning and five in the night), he acknowledges that "the amount of time is not as important as simply doing it daily." It could be hard to develop new habits, so if you start with five minutes a day, that's great. Feel free to sit or lie down, no matter what you feel most comfortable with.

What's the major connection between meditation and weight loss?

"Meditation can pose to be an important method to help people lose weight," Libshtein says. What exactly makes meditation so effective in this respect? It "aligns your conscious and unconscious mind with agreeing on changes that we want to make to our actions," he explains. These improvements may involve regulating food cravings and altering eating habits. It's crucial to get your unconscious mind involved because that's where unhealthy, weight-loss habits like emotional eating are entrenched. Meditation will help you become more conscious of these and, by practice, override them and even replace them with slimming habits.

Yet there's a more urgent reward for meditation. "Meditation can directly reduce stress hormone levels," Libshtein says. Stress hormones, such as cortisol, signal our bodies to store calories as fat. If you have so many cortisol flowing through your bloodstream, it will be hard to lose weight even if you make healthy choices. We know that sounds tough; we're all stressed out, and it seems difficult to shake.

Participants in the 2016 study showed "increased attention, relaxation, calmness, body-mind awareness, and brain activity" after just a few short sessions, according to Yi-Yuan Tang, Presidential Chair in Neuroscience and Professor the Department of Psychological Sciences at Texas Tech University. Your self-control can also increase with everyday practice, the study suggests. Researchers have successfully discovered that the parts of the brain most affected by meditation are those that help us to control ourselves. That means a few minutes of meditation a day will make it easier to move that second cookie or stop ice cream when you're feeling down.

How can meditation improve when diet and exercise don't seem to work?

"In many situations, stress is the primary cause for unnecessary weight gain or failure to lose weight," Libshtein states effectively. So, if you've been dieting and exercising, but you're always under stress, you may not be addressing the issue of holding your weight on. Again, stress releases hormones that store extra fat — what we don't want! This way can also fuel a stress cycle: you can't lose weight because you're stressed, which makes you stressed that you couldn't lose weight. It's an easy pattern to get trapped in; however, you can break it — and meditation can help you.

To properly deal with or remove stress, you first need to understand what triggers most anxiety in your life. Some stressors are easy to identify, but others may be more subtle. "I suggest using it to help you understand, track and cope with stress," says Libshtein. WellBe is a bracelet that acts a bit like a physical activity tracker, but it's the first of its kind to concentrate on mental health instead. Libshtein continues, "It also tells you who and what behaviors in your life cause emotional stress, so it can help you come up with new coping strategies that can help you lose weight."

How Do You Make Sure the Meditation Works for You?

If you want to add meditation to your weight-loss arsenal, it's crucial not to make it stressful. Meditation is intended to help you ditch the stress, not be a cause of stress. That's why we asked Libshtein for three simple ways to integrate a relaxing habit into your everyday life without feeling it's an extra task or a chore. You'll get the best results, of course, if you make meditation a routine and make time every day for even a few minutes of practice.

Use a mantra to help you lose weight.

A mantra is a word or phrase that you repeat to yourself to concentrate your practice and bring you back to the core when your mind wanders. As Libshtein states, "a mantra may give you something to concentrate on when you meditate." Although many people find it beneficial to practice it — especially if you choose something that resonates with you personally — it is absolutely unnecessary. Don't feel like you need to push yourself to use one if you don't feel normal or helpful. If you want to use one, Libshtein recommends you repeat it yourself as you inhale, and again as you exhale. Popular options include "I am cherished," "I am at ease," and "Om." If a mantra just doesn't sound right for you, Libshtein says it's just about your breathing.

Follow your breath to reduce your tension.

"Try using four counts for your inhalation and eight counts for your exhalation," Libshtein suggests. But meditation is all about minimizing tension, so if these counts sound strained or abnormal, it's okay to deviate from them. Try to raise your number every time you meditate. "Don't worry if it takes time for you to work up to eight counts," Libshtein says. "Just know that lengthening the exhalation will allow you to calm down."

Try a guided meditation on weight loss.

Feel lost on your own? There's no problem! There are many videos, podcasts, blogs, and phone apps that link you with experts who can direct you through meditation exercises before you feel comfortable going alone.

What do you expect from guided meditation for weight loss?

If you want to use meditation specifically to lose weight, look for guided meditations that concentrate on it as their subject. The expert in video or audio recording would probably ask you to imagine a few things: what you might look and sound like after you've lost weight, an inspirational person who's already managed to lose weight and what they might think and feel, what they might do to lose weight and get it off it, and how you can integrate these habits into your everyday lives.

Are there drawbacks to the use of weight loss meditation techniques?

Meditation can be used as only one method in the weight-loss toolkit. Diet and exercise are crucial aspects of the equation, too, and you're only going to get the best results when you incorporate all three of them into a long-term lifestyle. The secret to meditation, including food and exercise, is commitment. You need to stick to the practice to see positive improvements. "Research shows that meditation explicitly affects the structure of the brain after practicing for a prolonged period, such as 21 days," says Libshtein. That's why Mentors Channel is providing 21-day programs so that you can see improvements that really last.

How to Build A Room for Meditation in Your Home?

You will find it easier to stick to a meditation practice when you set yourself up for success. It can encourage your way to integrate meditation accessories and create a relaxing meditation space. Here's the equipment that will help you get started.

1. Essential Oil Distributor

Aromatherapy has been shown to have a soothing effect on the body, which is beneficial when you meditate. URPOWER's Essential Oil Diffuser lets you build a relaxing atmosphere so that you can enjoy the benefits of essential oils. Plus, the diffuser shuts off automatically when it runs out of the water, so that you can meditate for as long as you want, without any fear.

2. Bluetooth earphones

Don't you have enough room for a dedicated meditation space? You can carry these portable headsets anywhere you need to go. They're tiny, and they're synchronized with iPhones and Android devices, so you can listen to guided meditation anywhere without disturbing your family and friends.

3. Cotton Bolster Pillow Cushion

A floor pillow gives you a relaxing place to find your bliss, whether it's by yoga or meditation. Peace Yoga Zafu Meditation Yoga Buckwheat Filled Cotton Bolster Pillow Cushion relieves tension during long periods of sitting. Amazon reviewer Juli wrote, "In my yoga instructor training classes where we would sit (mostly) for 3 hours, I'd have a lot of hip pain trying to sit cross-legged. While raising my hips with a yoga block helped ease the pressure, it was not comfortable. This zafu is the ideal height and density to sit during class hours or practice meditation. "Bonus: the cover is machine-washable, so you can quickly clean the cushion.

What are the effects of weight loss meditation?

Meditation is not going to help you lose weight immediately. But with a little practice, it can potentially have long-lasting effects not just on your weight, but also on your thinking habits.

Durable weight loss

Meditation is related to a wide range of benefits. In terms of weight loss, mindfulness meditation appears the most beneficial. A 2017 study of current research showed that mindfulness meditation was a successful way of losing weight and improving eating habits.

Mindfulness meditation requires paying careful attention to the following:

- The place where you are
- What you are doing
- How you feel in the present moment

During mindfulness meditation, you can remember all of these things without judgment. Try to handle your acts and feelings just like those — nothing else. Take stock of what you feel and do, but try not to label something as good or bad. This fact is made simpler with daily practice.

Practicing mindfulness meditation can also contribute to long-term benefits. Compared to other diets, those practicing mindfulness are more likely to hold their weight off, according to the 2017 study.

Less guilt and shame

Mindfulness meditation can be especially useful in reducing emotional and stress-related eating. By becoming more conscious of your thoughts and feelings, you will notice the moments you eat because you are anxious, rather than hungry.

It's also a helpful method to keep you from slipping into the dangerous trap of shame and guilt that some people fall into when trying to improve their eating habits. Mindfulness meditation requires accepting your thoughts and actions for what they are, without judging yourself.

This way helps you to forgive yourself for making mistakes, such as eating a bag of potato chips. That forgiving will also keep you from catastrophizing, which is a fancy word for what happens when you decide to order a pizza because you've already "screwed up" by eating a bag of chips.

How Can I Start Meditating on Weight Loss?

Anyone who has a mind and a body should practice meditation. No special equipment or costly classes are required. For many, the most challenging part is just finding the time. Try to start with something fair, like 10 minutes a day or any other day.

During these 10 minutes, make sure you have access to a quiet spot. If you have children, you may want to cram them in until they wake up or go to bed to avoid interruption. You might also try to do it in the shower.

Once you're in a quiet place, make yourself comfortable. You can sit or lie down in any location that's easy to feel.

Start by concentrating on your breath, looking at your chest or stomach as it rises and falls. Feel the air as it passes in or out of your mouth or nose. Listen to the noises that the air is producing. Do this for a minute or two before you begin to feel more relaxed.

Next, with your eyes open or closed, follow the following steps:

1. Take a deep breath. Keep on for a few seconds.

2. Exhale and repeat slowly.

3. Breathe, of course.

4. Observe your breath when it reaches your nostrils, lifts your chest, or moves your abdomen, but do not change it in any way.

5. Continue to concentrate on your breath for 5 to 10 minutes.

6. You're going to find your mind wandering, which is natural. Just accept that your mind has drifted, and turn your attention back to your breath.

7. As you begin to wrap up, think about how quickly your mind has drifted. Then, remember how easy it was to put your focus back to your breath.

Try more days of the week than not to do this. Bear in mind that the first few times you do this may not feel very successful. But with daily practice, it's going to get easier and start to feel more normal.

Through my teaching experience, and through reading countless study papers, I have learned that the following are the best weight loss meditations.

1) Pranayama to increase the metabolic rate;

Pranayama is probably the best weight loss meditation ever. The term pranayama refers to the type of breathing that we do when practicing yoga. By incorporating yoga and meditation, we prepare the body and mind for fitness.

Scientific evidence indicates that people who practice a combination of meditation, yoga, and pranayama (breathing exercises used in yoga) have a higher BMR (Basal Metabolic Rate — the number of calories burned each period). An increased BMR rate allows us to lose weight more easily.

Some meditations are not suitable for weight loss because they are inactive, and inactivity triggers a decline in metabolic activity, which is counter-productive to slimming. On the other hand, according to the National Library of Medicine, pranayama will "acutely increase metabolism." In particular, Ujjayi Pranayama (filling the lungs by breathing through the nose) while performing Surya Anuloma Viloma (right nostril breathing) has been shown to increase oxygen intake by 19 percent due to increased muscle activity, and this, in turn, contributes to a higher metabolic rate.

While the research explicitly looked at the two approaches listed above, it does appear that other active meditations can also help with weight loss. That's why you would also like to try walking, tai chi, and kapalabhati.

2) Mindfulness Meditation Decreases Food Craving

Research shows that mindfulness meditation helps with weight loss by enhancing self-regulation and self-awareness and increasing executive function.

Mindfulness, in a nutshell, means being consciously mindful of the present moment in a non-judgmental way.

Whenever we are unaware of our thoughts and emotions, we allow them to guide us. If we say, "I like chocolate," if we're not aware of the concept, we're sure to grab a chocolate bar. `

Mindfulness gives us the power to say, "This is a thought. I don't want chocolate because I want to be smaller.

Only by becoming more conscious, we motivate ourselves to take control of our minds, which, in turn, allows us to take control of our actions.

One randomized controlled trial indicated that mindfulness meditation increased weight loss by 2.8 kg due to better eating habits and dietary restriction.

3. Visualization of weight loss

When it comes to weight loss, visualizations will help inspire you and make you feel good about getting in shape. Essentially, to create a weight loss visualization, we're building a mental picture of who we want to be. Then we're meditating on this photo. It's like you're meditating on the perfect image of yourself in all the glory of your bikini! And for your inspiration, it works wonders.

Data indicate that weight loss visualizations motivate us to kick dangerous habits. McGill University has studied how visualization improves our ability to regulate our diet. They asked the test participants to consume more fruit for a week. Half of the group were asked to imagine buying fruit and eating it at times and to write down a strategy to achieve their goal. The other half of the participants were in the control group. The findings of the analysis indicate that the test participants who conducted the study had twice as much fruit as the control group.

Try this quick visualization of weight loss:

1. Sit down gently for a few minutes and concentrate on your breathing.

2. Now, once you get in shape, imagine yourself. What will you be looking like? What would you like to feel? What's going to be different for you? Imagine these things in more depth

3. Now, tell yourself how you're going to get there. What are the steps you're taking to get in shape? Write down those steps.

4. Now imagine yourself going through the steps above before you hit the type of body you like.

5. Do this visualization once a day for a week every day.

4. Best Guided Weight Loss Meditation

Undoubtedly, you've seen the bajillion guided meditations for weight loss on YouTube. Some of them are fine. Some of them are suits. The strange few are genuinely extraordinary.

In my view, Michael Sealey is the best-guided meditation on weight loss. This way is called Hypnosis for Weight Loss

5. Visualization of weight loss

This way is a powerful weight loss meditation technique.

In this visualization, you are going to construct a very credible mental picture of the ideal.

You will see yourself as everything you want to be. You're going to train your mind to know what you want. This way is going to turbo-charge your slimming.

1) Sit comfortably in a comfortable spot. Make sure the spine is balanced correctly.

2) Close your eyes and take some minutes to concentrate on your breathing. Relax now.

3) It's a fun bit. You will systematically create a mental image of yourself as the person you want to be. And you're not going to dare go short on me. I want you to imagine yourself as being fantastic. I like your body to be the body you want. Everything is fine.

4) Start with your face. What the heck does your face look like? See your lovely skin. Note how nil wrinkles are. You look lovely. Vividly imagine the face.

5) The upper body. You might want a six-pack if you're a male. If you're just a kid, you might want a slim, slender look. Imagine the ideal upper body.

6) The legs: the tone? Smooth, huh? How are you going to want them? Imagine that in depth.

7) Anything else: please fill in all other specifics about your ideal body.

8) Imagine that this perfect you are doing something astounding-balls right now, something you'd have to get in shape to do. You might as well be crossing the finish line of a marathon. You could be standing on a stage with people staring at you. No matter what you wish, you could do, imagine it in depth.

9) Bring it together so that you can picture your dream self-fulfillment of something unique.

10) Affirmation: What would your ideal-self have said after achieving this impressive feat? Choose an affirmation, and imagine you say it clearly in your head.

11) It is important to imagine your ideal self in detail. You need to see your perfect body and honestly imagine that you will do that wonderful thing and hear the optimistic reinforcement in your mind.

6: Visualization of food assimilation

This way is a meditation on the topic of biological assimilation.

Biological assimilation is the mechanism by which the body breaks down nutrients and then assimilates them into the body.

Good food assimilation increases our overall well-being and helps us get in shape and stay fit.

Stress, however, impaired the body's ability to assimilate food, allowing the body to store more fat.

Meditation increases digestion by helping to assimilate food and reducing stress. However, we can take it further by visualizing the assimilation of food. In this meditation, we imagine the path of food through the body and its effect on us. This idea improves the mindfulness of body and food and, in turn, motivates us to eat healthier.

7: Mindfulness of feeding

Mindful eating is a game = changer for a lot of people.

Jean Kristeller [professor emeritus of psychology at Indiana State University] claims that mindfulness therapy has changed the way she thinks regarding slimming.

"It was more than just a moment of a light bulb," she said.

After hearing famous mindfulness instructor John Kabat Zinn talk about mindfulness, she decided to start a program called Mindfulness-Based Eating Awareness Training.

The curriculum helps people to be more conscious of food and the food process.

In one exercise, participants slowly consume a raisin while paying careful attention to the taste and the sensations of food.

"People are shocked at the workout," she says. "They see that if they eat a few raisins carefully, they will enjoy them as much or more than if they eat a whole package."

Mindful eating helps with diets because it makes you more conscious of the eating process. It enables you to understand how you feel about various types of food and what happens in your mind when you eat it. By becoming more conscious of the food processor, you are motivated to improve the process.

Directions

1. You'll need a piece of comfort food/dunk food that you still consume for this workout. It's your favorite.

2. Go to a quiet and peaceful place.

3. Place your fast food on the table/ground a few feet in front of you.

4. Sit back comfortably with a healthy stance.

5. Relax for a couple of minutes

6. Focus your mind on the feeling that your breath is coming and going through the gap between your nose and your mouth.

7. Take twenty-five thoughtful breaths.

8. Keep in mind your favorite junk food (the one that's in front of you).

9. Focus your attention on the perception of this food in your attention (do not look at the actual food, focus on the mental image of the food).

10. As you concentrate your mind on food, you will find that some thoughts are coming up. You're going to have clear food ideas. These are the thoughts that make up your negative relationship with food. We need to get rid of those feelings.

11. To get rid of your feelings, any time you encounter some thought, see the view (imagine that you're looking at yourself experiencing the idea as if you were looking at yourself). Next, say to yourself, "It is only a matter of course. It's not the truth.

12. Finally, imagine blowing the thought away from you until it disappears entirely.

13. Pick up your meal.

14. When you're holding the food in your lap, you'll feel different thoughts again.

15. Take a minute to note the kind of thoughts you're having.

16. Again, remind yourself that there are only emotions. They're not the reality; they're just the fantasies in your mind.

17. Now, to continue this exercise, I'm going to use the example of a chocolate bar, but you can continue with any food you have.

18. Open the chocolate bar, please. Search that. Meditate on it, guy. Focus your attention on the food, the colors, the scent, the texture, and every other element of the food.

19. Again, consider the kind of thoughts you're having. Tell yourself, "These are just feelings. They're not true. "Imagine those thoughts floating in the distance.

20. Eat your food slowly. Bite it in, keep it in your mouth, and stop. Then don't swallow it. Meditate on the taste.

21. Be mindful of your feelings with the food in your mouth. Tell yourself, "These are just feelings. They're not true. "Imagine the thoughts floating in the distance.

22. Swallow.

23. Keep eating until the food is finished.

By doing the weight loss meditation technique above, you're going to change your food thoughts.

You may have been shocked when I said that I would delete all thoughts, including positive reviews. You may have thought at one point (for example), "Food is nutrition. I'm expected to eat well. "This is a positive thought, isn't it? Then why do you get rid of it?

The reason to get rid of all the emotions, and not just the negative ones, is that there's a kind of mesh in the head. Thoughts are like an entangled piece of thread. Thinking of one good idea does not necessarily lead to another good view. If you think "I'm going to eat well," your next thought is just as likely to be "No, I probably won't because I have a poor diet" as "Yeah, I'm going to eat healthily and exercise."

Mental Exercise to Cut Calories and Learn to Avoid Temptations and Triggers

Here are nine ways to improve your attitude that will help you lose weight more healthily.

Check out what you know about weight loss.

Quora user Wilfredo Thomas argues that recognizing weight loss in the form of energy balance is the first key to the achievement of one's ideal body.

"Energy balance is a science-based way to say calories in versus calories out," he says. "The body needs a certain amount of calories to maintain its current body weight."

When you understand the energy balance, you can feel less inclined to eat more than you need.

Keep out of opaque food containers.

Neil O'Nova, the author of the novel, "7-Minute Skinny Jeans," warns against consuming food packages, boxes, and bags that are not plain.

"Our brains are highly visual. We take visual clues as to how much food we've consumed to help us know when we should stop," O'Nova says. "But when you can't see how much food you've eaten, you'll never get the visual input, and you'll end up overeating."

Measuring the portions and pouring them into a small bowl or a napkin will stop you from eating more than you had expected.

Ditch dieting.

O'Nova, too, is not a fan of conventional dieting since he believes that it restricts one's mind-set.

When you're out of your diet and losing weight, you can go back to eating badly, not exercising, and slowly gaining your pounds.

"Instead, concentrate on your long-term eating habits," he says. "This is the easiest way to lose weight and hold it off in a safe way."

Try to make your stomach feel whole.

O'Nova recommends you select vegetables such as carrots and celery over sweet treats when you have a snack craving.

Not only do they have fewer calories, but they're also fibrous and can make you feel stronger.

Think of exercise as an enjoyable activity.

Jared Haas, Supervisor of Geographic Information Systems, claims discovering a fun exercise is the essential thing, so you would be more able to integrate it into your weekly routine.

"If you hate running, don't run. It doesn't matter that running has been proven to help you lose weight," Haas writes. "If you dislike it too much, you're not going to stick with it. If you're not going to stick with it, it's not going to show lasting results."

Working with friends or in a group can be inspiring, making exercise less of a hassle and more fun after work or between assignments.

Understand what causes obesity to happen.

More cases of obesity are stated to be caused by lifestyle choices rather than by genetic factors.

Thomas points to a research study published online by the United States. The National Library of Medicine found that "promoting the notion of genes as a cause of obesity will increase genetically deterministic beliefs and minimize the incentive to participate in healthy lifestyle behaviors."

Thomas concludes that people who agree that unhealthful behaviors induce obesity are likely to become cautious and reconsider their actions.

Motivate yourself by posing some tough questions.

Although self-assertion can be beneficial, consider tapping into your competitive side by turning weight loss into a challenge.

"I find it a lot more motivating to challenge myself with self-talk like this: 'Will you lose this weight? Are you up to the challenge?'" writes O'Nova.

Be kind to yourself

Pharmacist and health enthusiast Noor Ullah Jan said, "You have to see yourself in a better light to get out of old propensities."

"Take a look at your future self, six months to a year not far out, and imagine how amazing you can look and sound," he says.

Get a bit more sleep.

"When we're sleep-deprived, high-fat and sugary food seems a lot more enticing, possibly because it gives us a fast burst of energy."

CONCLUSION

Experts believe that some diets that focus on reducing carbohydrates and increasing protein intake (meat) will contribute to weight loss. They claim, however, that there could be detrimental secondary effects over the long term. The Retaining medical chart supports this.

It states: low-carbohydrate diets, mainly when done without medical supervision, can be hazardous. They are engineered to induce rapid weight loss by fostering an undesirably high concentration of ketone bodies (a by-product of fat metabolism). If you are contemplating a low-carbohydrate diet, make sure to contact your doctor first. If you intend to lose weight, don't despair of winning. Weight management is not difficult, nor is it appropriate to mean starvation or a bland, repetitive diet. With deliberate effort and imagination, most people can effectively regulate their weight over the long term with a pleasant yet realistic diet and near-daily exercise. Longer, healthier life is undoubtedly worth the effort. Losing weight will come with your mind embracing the transition, and if you believe and work against the temptations and causes, you can achieve your goal of losing weight in less than ten days.

www.ingramcontent.com/pod-product-compliance
Lightning Source LLC
Chambersburg PA
CBHW070806240726

48654CB00007B/228